The Healthy Alternative

A Guide For A Pain-Free, Active Lifestyle

Dr. Todd P. Sullivan

ISBN: 978-1-4528157-5-6

PRINTED IN THE UNITED STATES OF AMERICA

Disclaimer
The contents of this book are for informational purposes only. It is sold with the understanding that the publisher and author are not engaged in rendering professional services to the reader. This book is not intended to be a substitute for professional medical advice, diagnosis, or treatment.

Every effort has been made to make this text as complete and accurate as possible. However, there may be errors, both typographical and in content. Furthermore, this book contains information that is only current up to the printing date. Due to the ever-changing nature of the subject matter, therefore, some of the research and materials contained may not represent the latest data available on the subject matter.

Always seek the advice of your physician or other qualified health provider with any questions you may have regarding a medical condition. Never disregard professional medical advice or delay in seeking it because of something you have read in this or any other book.

TABLE OF CONTENTS

INTRODUCTION

A s a child, I was always interested in becoming a doctor. I just did not know what type of doctor I wanted to become. In high school I played several sports and during one particular season when I was in high school, I injured my lower back. After going the traditional medical route for three weeks with no relief, my father said, *"Let's go to the family chiropractor."*

At that time, I had no clue what a chiropractor was or what they did. The following day, I went to the doctor's office, filled out my paperwork, and was taken into an exam room. I remember asking myself, *"Where are all the posters, pens, and brochures with the drug company and medication names on them? Why do all of the pictures on the wall have healthy messages on them?"* It was completely foreign, yet oddly comforting, to be in an office with such a healing atmosphere.

The doctor entered the room and asked me a series of questions about my problem. He then evaluated my movement, checked my reflexes, and explained to me that I had sprained my sacroiliac joint (SI joint). He showed me a spine model and some charts to help explain what was happening.

The doctor helped me to a table where I lay for 15 minutes with a heat pack and a machine with two pads that "massaged" my back. He put me through a series of slow and gentle stretches and laid me on my side. The area where I had hurt for over three weeks made a small "popping" sound, and like an immediate release of pressure, my pain was gone. The doctor showed me three stretches I could do at home and explained to me how I could avoid a relapse.

No pills. No needles. No surgery I remember thinking this chiropractic care is great. My pain was gone immediately and, to my excitement, did not return. Because the problem had been explained to me, I was armed with the knowledge of what was wrong and what could be done for it and how I could prevent injuring myself while maintaining an active lifestyle.

After finishing my undergraduate education and receiving my Bachelor of Science degree, my interest in the workings of the human body, diet, exercise, combined with my enjoyment of problem solving and a desire to help people, culminated in the pursuit of a career as a Doctor of Chiropractic. Chiropractic care had made such a big difference in my life that I wanted to dedicate my life to it.

I am a Doctor of Chiropractic because I honor the inborn potential of everyone to be truly healthy. I wish to **assist** with healing rather than *intrude*—to free rather than control. I choose to care for the <u>patient</u> with the disease, <u>not</u> care for the disease. Every day, I am confronted with painful and challenging spinal syndromes. Every day, I am able to see miracles and offer hope.

This book is about learning about the wonders of the human body and the fact that the nervous system is the master controller of every system in the body. It is about understanding the medical fact that a body of growing evidence suggests that many conditions can be traced back to spinal dysfunction.

When confronted with back or neck pain, *The Healthy Alternative: A Guide For A Pain-Free, Active Lifestyle* involves understanding your treatment options and integrating the safest, most effective ways to manage and prevent pain. By using the right formula of conventional treatment methods (medication, injections, pain management techniques, etc.) as well as more conservative options (diet, exercise, chiropractic, etc.), you can solve your own problems and regain and maintain a healthy spine and nervous system.

The literal meaning of the word "doctor" is "educator." The goal of this book is to share life-changing lessons with you and help to clear up any confusion in an ever-changing health care environment. My hope is that these lessons will serve to teach you to understand true health and to live free of pain.

Each of the book's eight chapters cover important topics that are relevant to your health. In the first chapter, you will learn the basics of how your body works. This may be the most important chapter in the whole book because the better you understand how the body works, the better health choices you can make. The remaining chapters include information about back and neck pain, headaches and whiplash injuries, as well as a variety of diagnostic and therapeutic options that are available to help you manage or completely eliminate your pain.

CHAPTER 1

The Human Body

"The human body represents the actions of three laws: spiritual, mechanical and chemical, united as one triune. As long as there is a perfect union of these three, there is health."

D.D. Palmer, the founder of chiropractic

When you sit calmly reading this, your body is bristling with activity. The trillions of cells that make up your body are busy at work performing thousands of delicately balanced processes that make your life possible. The brilliance with which your body controls this profoundly complex dance of chemistry is truly awe-inspiring. As long as your body is able to keep the dance going, you remain healthy and vibrant. However, if there is a disruption in any of the body's processes, the entire system loses its ability to perform correctly and disease emerges.

Such is the miracle of life. Our anatomy is the structure that makes up our body's assets, while our physiology is the infinite amount of interrelated functions our body processes to keep us adapting to our ever-changing environment. **Having a good understanding of and an appreciation for your anatomy and physiology can help you create a new level of confidence and trust in yourself and your body.** The best way for you to build your health is to understand the assets of your body and know how to best protect them each and every day.

The body's ability to regulate and control the delicate balance of all of life's necessary processes is called "homeostatis." The term homeostatis is derived from the Greek words for "same" and "steady." It refers to the way the body acts to maintain a stable internal balance. For example, your body works to maintain a carefully regulated internal temperature of 98.6 degrees. If you go outside on a warm day and begin to work, your body will begin to sweat in an effort to keep your temperature stable. You may also begin to breathe deeper in an effort to keep your tissues supplied with oxygen during a period of increased demand, such as during intense exercise.

Disease and disability result whenever the body is stressed beyond its ability to maintain homeostasis. This stress can come from several sources including interference or irritation of the nervous system, trauma, poor diet, lack of exercise, or excessive emotional stress. In this chapter, you will learn about the systems in your body that are necessary for maintaining health.

DIGESTIVE SYSTEM

When we eat such things as bread, meat, and vegetables, they are not in a form that the body can use. Everything that we eat and drink must be broken down into smaller molecules before they can be absorbed and used by the body. This process is called digestion.

The digestive system includes the digestive tract and its accessory organs, which process food into molecules that can be absorbed and utilized by the cells of the body. Food is broken down, bit by bit, until the molecules are small enough to be absorbed and the waste products are eliminated. The digestive tract, also called the alimentary canal or gastrointestinal (GI) tract, includes the mouth, esophagus, stomach, small intestine, and large intestine.

As long as this system works correctly, the nutrients you consume can be extracted and absorbed into the blood stream to be delivered to your individual cells. The digestive system is the means by which you get all of the individual nutrients that are needed for health. Every single molecule in your entire body arrived there in the same way—at some point in the recent past you ate it. This is an important concept to remember because if your diet does not include everything that your body needs, you will lose some of the richness of your health. Consuming food is much like depositing money into your checking account. If you don't have enough resources there, you can't afford to keep fixing your house.

CARDIOVASCULAR SYSTEM

The cardiovascular system is sometimes called the circulatory system. It consists of the heart, which is a muscular pumping device, and a closed system of vessels called arteries, veins, and capillaries. The role of the cardiovascular system in maintaining homeostasis is the transportation of nutrients and oxygen from the digestive system to all of the cells in the body, as well as the transportation of waste and carbon dioxide to the be eliminated.

As long as your cardiovascular system works correctly, your body has an enormous capacity to adapt to just about any external demand. For example, when you begin to exercise, your heart pumps fast and your blood pressure increases in order to supply more oxygen and nutrients to your tissues. When you are cold, your blood vessels constrict in some areas of the body—the back of your arm, for instance—in an effort to conserve heat. When you body is injured, the blood vessels open up to allow white blood cells to enter the area to fight infection and speed healing.

Unfortunately, the cardiovascular system is the one that fails most often due to an unhealthy lifestyle. Heart disease is the number one cause of death in the United States and is also responsible for tragic disabilities in millions of Americans. The vast majority of heart disease is completely avoidable by making some simple lifestyle changes—exercise being the most important. **The key phrase when it comes to your cardiovascular health is "use it or lose it."** If you don't exercise and work out your cardiovascular system, you will lose it.

IMMUNE SYSTEM

Every minute of the day, we are exposed to dangerous bacteria, viruses, fungi, and the development of cancerous cells that, if allowed to grow, would result in illness or death. In fact, the bacteria and viruses living in and on our body outnumber our own cells. What keeps these invaders in check is the immune system.

When your immune system is compromised due to improper diet, stress, or trauma, lack of exercise, spinal disorders, or for any other reason, you lose some of your ability to eliminate harmful cells and invaders in your body, resulting in disease. Just like with your body's other systems, your lifestyle choices have a profound impact on how well your immune system functions.

THE NEUROMUSCULOSKELETAL SYSTEM

The neuromusculoskeletal system is really three distinct systems that work as one coordinated unit:

1. The bones and joints (skeletal system)
2. The muscles
3. The nervous system

The neuromusculoskeletal system is by far the largest system in the body, comprising between 60%-70% of your total body mass. It is also the most prone to injuries, dysfunction, and pain. Understanding how each of these systems work will provide you with the information to make better treatment and lifestyle choices and to live your life free from pain and disability.

THE BONES AND JOINTS

The human skeleton is made up of more than 200 bones that are connected by joints. Your bones are responsible for creating your body's general shape, and they serve to protect your internal organs and to manufacture blood cells. Each of your bones is made up of two compounds: a protein meshwork of collagen and a salt of calcium called hydroxyapatite.

The collagen fibers that make up the basic structure of your bones, give them a great deal of resilience and resistance to breaking when twisted, bent, or impacted. It is actually the loss of this collagen meshwork and not just a loss of calcium that is responsible for the bone weakness associated with conditions such as osteoporosis. The other component of bone, hydroxyapatite, is a crystalline calcium salt, which is integrated into the collagen meshwork. Hydroxyapatite is responsible for giving the bones rigidity and resistance to crushing under pressure.

Bones can be compared to steel-reinforced concrete, where the collagen acts much like the steel meshwork in the concrete, and the hydroxyapatite acts much like the concrete that surrounds the steel. Together they form a very tough, resilient, and rigid framework upon which the rest of the body is supported. Because your bones are rigid and do not bend, you would not be able to move if it were not for your joints.

Joints are much more than simply a place where the ends of two bones meet. They are very complicated systems of ligaments, tendons, membranes, fluid, and cartilage that allow the bones to move in a smooth, stable, and controlled way. Joints are designed in a wide variety of ways depending on their function and the particular stresses they have to endure. For example, the joints between the sternum (breastbone) and your ribs are simple joints consisting only of fibrous collagen. They are designed to be simple because the front part of your rib cage does not have to move very much in relation to your sternum. The shoulder joint, on the other hand, is an extremely complex joint that requires a whole host of muscles, ligaments, and tendons all working in concert with each other in order to move properly. If any one of the muscles or other structures of the shoulder are damaged, pain, instability, or loss of function may result.

MUSCLES

There are more than 650 muscles in your body that have only one purpose—to create movement. **While your bones are what give your body its framework, the muscles are what give your body motion.** There is more than three times the number of muscles in your body as there are bones, and each one of these muscles fills a particular role in creating movement. Like bones, your muscles also contain a lot of collagen for strength and resilience. Instead of calcium salts, muscles contain a specialized type of cell, which has the unique ability to contract when stimulated by the nervous system.

There are actually three types of muscles in the body—smooth muscle, cardiac muscle, and striated muscle (also called skeletal muscle). Smooth muscle is found surrounding the organs of the digestive tract as well as the arteries. In the digestive tract, smooth muscle is responsible for moving the food we eat through our digestive system, while the smooth muscle, which surrounds the arteries, helps the regulation of blood flow throughout the body. Unlike skeletal muscles, smooth muscles are involuntary muscles, meaning that we do not have conscious control over them.

Cardiac muscle, as its name implies, is found only in the heart. What differentiates cardiac muscle from all other muscle in the body is the fact that it rhythmically contracts on its own, regardless of stimulation by the nervous system. As a matter of fact, if two independent cardiac cells, each rhythmically contracting to their own beat, are put in contact with each other, they will begin beating in unison.

The third type of muscle is the skeletal muscle. This is the type of muscle that we can consciously control and the type of muscle that is of most interest to us because it is the type of muscle responsible for our posture and movement. Every skeletal muscle attaches to at least two different bones. As they contract, they draw the bones together using the joints as hinges.

Take for example the elbow joint. Compared to some of the other joints in the body such as the shoulder or hip, the elbow is a relatively simple hinge joint. Yet there are more than a dozen muscles, which cross the elbow joint, all of which contribute to the elbow's normal movement. If any of these muscles do not fire in a highly coordinated fashion, or if some of the muscles are tighter or weaker than they should be, abnormal joint function and pain will likely result.

Abnormal posture and joint motion resulting from weak, spastic, or uncoordinated muscles is very common, especially in people who work at a desk all day. Since muscles become weaker unless they are exercised, it is important for good muscular health to include some form of resistance exercise as part of your daily routine.

THE NERVOUS SYSTEM— "THE MASTER CONTROL CENTER"

The nervous system is made up of trillions of highly specialized individual nerve cells, each of which communicate with hundreds or thousands of other nerve cells through tiny electrical pulses, and is comprised of two major systems. The first is the central nervous system, which includes your brain and spinal cord, and the other is called the peripheral nervous system, which includes the nerves that run from your spine to all areas of the body.

The nervous system is called the master control center, as it is responsible for the control of all major body functions including our senses, movement and balance, as well as the regulation of all body functions.

There are three types of nerves: pain, or sensory nerves, motor nerves, and postural nerves, or more correctly, proprioceptors. Pain nerves do just what their name implies—they allow us to feel pain. Whenever something in our body hurts, it is because the pain nerves in the area are being stimulated and are sending signals to the brain to create the sensation of pain.

Motor nerves are responsible for controlling movement by stimulating muscles to contract. The fact that you are able to hold this book in your hands right now is because these motor nerves are contracting the muscles in your hands and arms. If these nerves aren't able to function correctly, it can result in weakness or paralysis in the muscles they control.

The third type of nerve is the proprioceptors, or what we will simply call the postural nerves. These nerves are responsible for sending information to the brain about where your body is and what it's doing. For example, if you close your eyes and hold your arm out to your side, you can tell exactly where your arm is even though you can't see it because the postural nerves of the arm and upper back tell the brain where your arm is. Many people have discovered what happens when their postural nerves aren't working correctly after they have had too much to drink. Alcohol partially disrupts the function of your cerebellum and postural nerves, making it difficult to touch your finger to your nose when your eyes are closed or walk a straight line with your eyes open.

THE SPINE

The human spine is a column of up to 34 bones called vertebrae, separated by tough fibrous pads called discs (or intervertebral discs).

The spine is divided into five areas: the top seven vertebrae make up the cervical region (neck); below the neck are twelve thoracic vertebrae to which your twelve pairs of ribs attach; the low back region is made up of five lumbar vertebrae; below the lumbar region, there are five fused vertebrae that make up the sacrum; and finally, at the very base of the spine is the group of three fused vertebrae called the coccyx. On the other side of the sacrum are the two bones of the pelvis.

THE SPINAL VERTEBRAE

Each vertebra consists of a vertebral body, which is a large oval-shaped solid block of bone, and a vertebral arch, which is located on the back of the vertebral body and creates the space through which the spinal cord runs. The vertebral body provides about 70% of all the structural support of the spine.

THE SPINAL CANAL AND VERTEBRAL ARCH

Directly in back of the vertebral body is an opening called the spinal canal. When all of the bones are stacked on top of each other, one continuous canal is formed. This is where the spinal cord runs from the brain down to all of the areas of the body.

Surrounding the spinal canal is the bony vertebral arch. Attached to the arch is a pair of joints called facet joints, and three body protrusions called processes. The facet joints act as links holding the vertebrae together and strengthening the spine. They also bear 30% of the structural support of the spine.

The process located in the center of the arch is called the spinous process. These are the bony bumps that you can feel running down the center of your back. On either side of the spinous process are the two transverse processes. The processes act as anchor points for ligaments and muscles necessary for movement.

THE FACET JOINTS

The facet joints play a large role in restricting the way in which two adjacent vertebra move in relation to each other. For example, in the cervical spine (neck), the facet joints are oriented in such a way as to allow a considerable degree of rotation, whereas the facet joints in the lumbar spine (low back) are oriented in a way that restricts rotation. A simple experiment of turning your head from side to side and then trying to twist your lower back to the same degree shows the effect facet joints have on the movement of the spine.

THE INTERVERTEBRAL DISCS

Each vertebra is attached to two adjacent spinal vertebrae with a disc between them. These discs, technically called intervertebral discs, are thick pads of fibrocartilage that act as shock absorbers and give the spine its ability to flex and twist. The disc itself is kind of like a jelly-filled donut. It has an outer fibrous portion called the annulus, and a soft jelly-like center called the nucleus pulposis.

THE SPINAL CORD

The spine forms the protective housing for the spinal cord, which begins at the brain stem (back of the skull) and extends like a wire down the length of the spine. Ultimately, the spinal cord sends out nerve branches that send and receive signals to and from every cell in the body. The close relationship between the spine and the spinal cord means that damage to any of the discs or vertebrae can also affect the spine or portion of the spinal cord associated with it, causing pain or abnormal function of the structures innervated by the affected area.

Between each pair of vertebrae and behind the disc, there is a small space where the nerves exit from the spinal cord and run to all of the areas of the body. These spaces are called the vertebral foramen. Foramen is a medical term that simply means "hole."

THE LIGAMENTS

Tough, flexible bands of fiber called ligaments help to hold the joints in the spine together. In conjunction with the facet joints, the ligaments help to keep the spine in one piece. There are four long ligaments that run down the entire length of the spine, as well as ligaments around each facet joint. Joint movement is important to keep the ligaments from becoming stiff. For this reason, regular physical activity is important to ensure that your maintain flexibility in the spine.

THE MUSCLES

Muscles attach to the bony extensions of the vertebrae and provide movement in the spine by contracting in a highly coordinated way. Muscles tend to work in pairs, each pulling the bones across a joint in the opposite direction, and are important for stabilizing and strengthening the spine, as well as providing movement. Like ligaments, muscles are also important for absorbing shock and releasing it in a controlled way.

FUNCTIONS OF THE SPINE

The spine is designed to do four things simultaneously: 1) to protect the spinal cord that serves as the primary communication conduit between your brain and the rest of your body; 2) to serve as a structural support and attachment for muscles and ligaments; 3) to provide mobility and flexibility to allow you to bend forward to touch your toes, swim, throw a baseball, and turn your head; and 4) the spine is responsible for transmitting body weight when walking and standing. Unfortunately, with this degree of mobility and flexibility comes potential instability and susceptibility to injury.

PROTECTION

Your spinal cord is a very soft and delicate bundle of nerves linking the communication between the brain and the rest of the body. Any damage to the spinal cord can result in devastating disabilities. One of the important roles of the spine is to encase the spinal cord in a strong bony structure for protection.

STRUCTURE

When viewed from the front or back, the spine should appear perfectly straight and symmetrical, reflecting the fact that your body is also symmetrical when viewed from the front or back. When viewed from the side, however, three major curves should be seen—one in each of the cervical, thoracic, and lumbar regions. These are the called "lordotic" curves. Next, the curves in the thoracic region bend forward. These are called "kyphotic" curves. As strange as it may seem, these curves actually add a considerable amount of strength and resiliency to the spine. Think about the curves as being like a spring, allowing the spine to flex and absorb shock much better than if it were straight. When a region of the spine loses its normal curve, the discs that separate the vertebrae can begin to degenerate and joints in that area can become less mobile.

MOVEMENT

The spine is not just a rigid support system for the rest of the body. Its design is essential to your ability to walk, run, lift, reach, climb, or perform any other activity. To allow this great degree of movement, the spine must be very flexible. However, this flexibility comes with an increased risk of injury. This is why the areas of the spine that have the greatest degree of flexibility—the neck and low back—are the most likely to become injured, while the areas with the most stability—the skull, thoracic spine, and the sacrum—are less prone to injury.

A HEALTHY SPINE

To achieve a healthy back, every part of the spine—the bones, joints, discs, ligaments, muscles, and nerves—must all work in unison, each contributing to stability, power, movement, strength, and flexibility. Often, we go about our daily activities without worrying about back pain. But when we suffer from back pain, we are reminded of just how important a healthy spine is to our quality of life. With the right treatment and regular care, our spines can remain strong and health throughout our lives.

CHAPTER 2

Low Back Pain

"Nobody in America should be allowed to have back surgery unless they have seen a chiropractor first."

Robert Mendelsohn, M.D.

Low back pain is very common in the United States. In fact, eighty percent of all people suffer from back pain at some point in their lives. Back pain is the second most common reason for visits to the doctor's office, outnumbered only by upper-respiratory infections. It has been estimated that low back pain affects more than half of the adult population each year, and more than 10% of all people experience frequent bouts of low back pain.

The susceptibility of the low back to injury and pain is due to the fact that the low back, like the neck, is a very unstable part of the spine, unlike the thoracic spine, which is supported and stabilized by the rib cage. This instability allows us to have a great deal of mobility, but it comes at the cost of increased risk of injury.

As long as it is healthy and functioning correctly, the low back can withstand tremendous forces without injury. Professional power lifters can pick up several hundred pounds off the floor without injuring their low back. However, if the low back is not moving properly or has weakened supporting muscles, something as simple as taking a bag of groceries out of the trunk of the car, picking something off the floor, or even simply bending down to pet the dog can cause a low back injury.

Until recently, researchers believed that back pain would heal on its own. We have learned, however, that is not always true. Recent studies showed that when back pain is left untreated, it may go away temporarily but will most likely return. For this reason, it is important to seek care with a qualified practitioner when back or neck pain occurs or when you experience an injury. Chiropractors who focus to prevent reoccurrence often successfully manage low back problems before they become chronic.

THE CAUSES OF LOW BACK PAIN

As we talked about earlier, the back is a complicated structure of bones, joints, discs, ligaments, and muscles. You can sprain ligaments, strain muscles, rupture disks, develop trigger points, and irritate joints, all of which can lead to back pain. While sports injuries or accidents can lead to injury and pain, sometimes even the simplest movements, like picking up a pencil off the floor, can have painful results. In addition, conditions such as arthritis, poor posture, obesity, psychological stress, kidney stones, kidney infections, blood clots, tumors, or bone loss can also lead to low back pain.

Due to the fact that there are so many things that can cause low back pain and some of those things can be quite serious if left untreated, it is important to seek professional help. Chiropractors are experts at diagnosing the cause and determining the proper treatment for low back pain. In this next section, we will address the most common causes of back pain.

THE INTERVERTEBRAL DISC

As we previously discussed, the intervertebral disc is a spongy pad that separates the vertebrae of the spine, creating a shock-absorbing cushion. Most experts agree that the disc is one of the most common sources of back pain. The center of the disc, called the nucleus, is made of a gel-like material. This nucleus is surrounded by annular fibers that encircle and contain the nucleus. These fibers are arranged much like a series of rubber bands and are designed to contain the nucleus.

DEGENERATIVE DISC DISEASE

Beginning in our teens, the intervertebral disc begins to lose some of the fluid. During this dehydration process, the disc is receiving less nutrition, slowly causing the disc to lose its ability to resist compression; and the space where the disc lies begins to lose its height.

When the space begins to narrow due to a loss of fluid within the disc, problems can occur. Degenerative disc disease is the term used by health care providers to describe this process. On an x-ray, this often shows up as a loss of the normal space between vertebrae. More specific tests, such as an MRI, may show a loss of water content and dehydration, narrowing of the holes where the spinal nerves exit (known as foramen), and ripping of the layers of cartilage (called annular tears) in the outer portion of the disc. Although these findings can be seen with people without any symptoms, the loss of disc space and fluid, and the associated pathology, can cause significant pain and disability.

DISC INJURIES

When the nucleus of an intervertebral disc loses its fluid, the normal motion of the spine at that level is lost. The resulting abnormality can cause tearing or ripping of the outer portion of the disc. This may result in a series of events that allow the nucleus to push its way through the outer annulus, putting pressure on the spinal nerve roots. This essentially "chokes" the nerve and often results in severe pain, burning, or numbness in the low back, buttocks, or legs.

Often, it is difficult for the person with disc problems to sit for very long, as this increases the pressure within the disc. Standing, too, may be difficult, and when a person with a severe disc problem stands up, they often cannot straighten into a full erect standing position. Many times, they lean to one side or another, which is the body's way of protecting the nerve from being compressed further.

A bulging, protruded, or slipped disc occurs when the inner nucleus pushes on the outer annulus fibers of the disc, pressing on spinal nerves.

A ruptured or herniated disc occurs when the nucleus pushes through the outer fibers of the disc and leaks into the spinal foramen or canal, irritating the spinal nerves by direct pressure or an inflammatory reaction. Leg pain, numbness, burning, tingling, or weakness is often the unfortunate result.

Although disc problems may be diagnosed by history and physical examination, an MRI scan best shows disc disorders and will confirm the diagnosis.

Despite the severity of pain often associated with a disc disorder, most cases of disc problems respond very well to conservative chiropractic treatments. Spinal decompression and chiropractic adjustments are often useful in relieving the pain, reducing disc protrusion, and restoring movement to irritated or inflamed joints that surround disc problems.

Spinal decompression therapy has been shown to be effective in cases of bulging and herniated discs. This technique, which is discussed later in Chapter 5, is aimed at decreasing pressure within the disc. Exercises from your chiropractor, such as The McKenzie Method, and core stabilization exercises, may help reduce pain and allow for rehabilitation of the region.

In about 2% of disc cases, surgery will be necessary to remove the disc or decompress the nerve exit area.

FACET SYNDROME

Facet joints disorders are some of the most common of all the recurrent spinal problems. The spinal facet joints are found at every spinal level and provide about 20% of the torsional (twisting) motion and stability in the back. These joints stabilize the spine while allowing for flexibility and protection of the spinal nerves. Each facet joint is positioned in the spine at a specific angle to provide the needed limits and ease of motion as to prevent slippage of one vertebra over another.

Facet joints are in almost perpetual motion. Because of this, these spinal joints may wear out and become degenerated. This process is not age-related and can occur to anyone at any time. When the facet joints become worn down, the cartilage within them may become thin or disappear, resulting in pain and decreased motion.

Each facet joint is coated by a very low friction moist cartilage and is surrounded by a capsule that has a rich supply of nerves, as well as a sticky fluid lubricant for the joint. This fluid, known as synovial fluid, may become less viscous and turn from an egg white consistency to that of chicken fat. Small pieces of joint cartilage, called synovial tags or meniscoids, may become trapped within the joint, causing severe pain with certain movements. This sets the stage for pain- limited motion, and interference with normal daily activities.

Symptoms of facet joint problems are often unpredictable. Usually, there are several episodes over a period of time. In many cases, pain may be very localized over the involved joint. It is rare that a facet injury causes pain or numbness in the leg, but the pain can radiate into the buttocks, groin, and thigh. In an attempt to protect the injury, muscles often go into spasm around the joint. This spasm will often be painful as well (*see "Sprains, Strains, and Spasm" section*). Typically, facet syndrome pain will become much worse when a person bends backwards or rotates to one side.

Although common, facet syndrome is not always easy to diagnose, and several other problems (abdominal tumors, spinal fractures, kidney stones, etc.) need to be ruled out by your doctor before the diagnosis is confirmed. Chiropractors are well-trained in the process of differentially diagnosing this problem through not only physical examination, but other tests such as x-rays, blood-work, or urinalysis when necessary to exclude serious pathology. Although well-trained in hands-on diagnosis, therapists like massage therapists, physical therapists, or occupational therapists, do not have the training or ability to order tests that may help them confirm what they think is wrong.

Fortunately, facet syndrome can often be effectively managed without surgery or the prolonged use of drugs. Chiropractic adjustment is the treatment that has been the most prescribed for pain that is coming from the facet joints. Spinal adjustments, combined with exercise, often help individuals gain relief and prevent or minimize recurrences of facet syndrome.

VERTEBRAL SUBLUXATION

The vertebral subluxation is a group of symptoms that can arise when one vertebra has lost its normal function and position in relation to the one above or below it. Subluxation can be seen anywhere in the spinal column and can be responsible for dysfunction in the lower back, mid-back, or neck. Put simply, a subluxation is a disruption in the normal movement of a spinal segment that can result in pain, inflammation, nerve irritation, and loss of normal function.

I often refer to subluxation as a "low-grade facet syndrome." Before a spinal problem becomes advanced, and sometimes before symptoms even occur, slight distorations, malrotations, or misalignments of the spine can occur secondary to poor posture, scoliosis or cogential disorders, injury, muscular incoordination, or early spinal degenerative disc or joint disease. With trauma or advanced arthritis, subluxation can become more insidious and painful.

Chiropractors are the only professionals who are trained to diagnosis and treat what are called spinal subluxations. The word *subluxation* comes from the Latin words meaning, "to dislocate" and "somewhat" or "slightly". So, the term vertebral subluxation literally means: "a slight misalignment of the bones in the spine."

Although the term was adequate in the 1800s when much was still misunderstood about the human body, today the word "subluxation" has changed in meaning to include the complex neurological, structural, and functional changes that occur when a spinal joint is not moving properly. For this reason, chiropractors usually refer to a chiropractors usually refer to a subluxation of the spine as a "Vertebral Subluxation Complex" or "VSC" for short. There are actually five components that contribute to subluxation:

1. **Spinal kinesiopathology:** This is the "bone and joint" component of subluxation and is seen when a vertebra is out of position, not moving properly, or has undergone degeneration. Physical stress, emotional stress, or chemical stress may

also cause this problem. With altered joint mechanics, there is loss of normal bending, turning, or other movements.

2. **Neuropathophysiology:** When spinal biomechanics are altered, there is a disruption of the normal messages traveling along the nerve fibers, which are often pinched, twisted, choked, stretched, distorted, or otherwise irritated by abnormal spinal function. This may result in numbness, tingling, or pain in the area of dysfunction or anywhere along the course of the irritated nerve. The result can be distorted signals from the brain to the nerve's target area, and subsequent dysfunction.

3. **Myopathology:** Since nerves exiting the spine control the muscles that help stabilize the vertebrae, the muscular component is an integral part of subluxation. When there is abnormal spinal movement, certain spinal support muscles may weaken or atrophy (shrink). Other muscles around the subluxation may go into spasm to protect the injured or dysfunctional spinal segment. A viscous cycle ensues, as muscle spasms pull the vertebrae further out of normal position. Spinal muscular support will be difficult or impossible as muscular tissue becomes fibrotic and produces scar tissue or when it becomes weak and atrophies. Lack of muscular coordination can contribute to bulging or herniated discs, which may place pressure on nerve roots or the spinal cord itself.

4. **Histopathology:** Subluxation can also affect the tendons, ligaments, and other soft tissues surrounding the spine. Swelling and inflammation can cause these soft tissues to become painful or easily torn, stretched, or scarred, leaving the spine with instability or restriction. Spinal instability from poor ligament strength can cause the body to stabilize the subluxation early, by depositing calcium, which can be seen as bony spurs on an x-ray.

5. **Pathophysiology:** Poorly functioning spinal joints often change the local chemistry in that area of the spine. As early as 1969, studies have repeatedly shown inflammatory chemicals such as phospholipase A2, as well as an acidic pH, to be present in the spinal nerves. When these chemicals are released, they can cause chemical inflammation and irritation of the tissues and nerves in that region of the spine, including areas where the inflamed nerve extends.

These changes may get progressively worse over time if they are not treated correctly, leading to chronic pain, inflammation, arthritis, muscle trigger points, the formation of bone spurs, loss of range of motion, as well as muscle weakness and spasms. Chiropractors have known the dangers of subluxation ever since the birth of the profession. More and more, scientific research is demonstrating the impact that subluxations have on the various tissues of the body.

In order to be truly healthy, it is vital for your nervous system to be functioning free of interference from subluxations. Spinal subluxations can often be detected by feeling the area—known as palpation—reading x-rays, or doing a postural analysis. **Chiropractors are the only health professionals trained in the detection, locations, and correction of the subluxation.**

SCIATICA

Sciatica is not a cause of low back pain, but is a non-specific term referring to pain, burning, or numbness in the buttock or leg.

The sciatica nerve is the largest nerve in the body. This nerve exits the spine and runs through your hip area and buttocks and down each leg. The sciatic nerve then branches into smaller nerves as it travels down the leg, providing feeling to your thighs and legs. It also controls the muscles in your legs and feet.

Sciatica is a sign that there is an underlying problem putting pressure on the nerve. The nerve can be pinched, mechanically compressed, or inflamed anywhere along its course from the spine to the toes. Sciatica is seen in all age groups but is most common in people between the ages of 30 and 50.

Most commonly, the sciatic nerve is compressed by a disc problem (bulges, protrusions, or herniations of disc material) in your lower back. These cases often resolve with non-surgical treatment such as spinal decompression, chiropractic adjustments, physiotherapy modalities, and home exercises.

In very rare cases of sciatic nerve compression with a serious condition known as cauda equine syndrome, the legs may become progressively weak, and bowel or bladder incontinence can occur. This is a medical emergency and usually requires immediate medical attention and probably surgery.

Piriformis syndrome is a condition that occurs when the sciatic nerve is compressed or entrapped as it runs through the piriformis muscle, which is located in the buttock area. As this is a muscular problem, surgery is never prescribed for this syndrome. Often, a course of Active Release Techniques, as discussed in Chapter 7, and home stretches will solve the pain associated with Piriformis syndrome.

SPINAL STENOSIS

Stenosis is a term used by health professionals to describe a narrowing of any opening or hole within the body. You may have heard of arterial stenosis, a condition where the arteries that carry blood flow away from the heart are blocked or narrowed by plaques or fatty deposits.

As the term implies, spinal stenosis is a narrowing of the spinal foramen or canal that results in the compression of the nerves that exit the spine to control the body. Just as a narrowed artery will not give adequate blood supply to the organ it transports blood to, a narrowed spinal canal or nerve opening can result in pain, weakness, or poor neural supply to its targeted body parts.

There are two types of spinal stenosis: foraminal stenosis and canal stenosis. Foraminal stenosis is a narrowing of the small foramen, or hole, that a single spinal nerve passes through after it exits the safety of the bony spinal canal. This compression, which is often due to bulging discs, bony spurs, subluxation, or facet joint arthritis, is usually associated with pain, burning, or numbness along the route of one spinal nerve. A doctor who is well trained in diagnosis is often able to localize the nerve involved by checking the patient's sensation along specific nerve root paths or tapping specific reflexes.

Spinal stenosis, on the other hand, is a more "generalized" narrowing. With spinal stenosis, the entire spinal opening for the spinal cord (called the spinal canal) is decreased. The causes of spinal stenosis are the same as those seen with foraminal stenosis, but because the entire spinal cord (and not one specific nerve) is compressed, symptoms are often felt in both legs. In many cases of spinal stenosis, patients feel better when they bend forward (which has been shown to increase the diameter of the spinal canal), and feel worse after a long walk or when they bend backwards (as this often narrows the space available for the spinal cord within the canal).

DEGENERATIVE JOINT DISEASE

Degenerative Joint Disease is sometimes known as "spinal arthritis" or "spondylosis." I like to refer to this condition as spinal decay, because just like your teeth decay your spine can essentially decay as well. Many of my patients who have already had x-rays or an MRI tell me that they have "arthritis" in their spine. Often the significance of spinal arthritis is downplayed by other doctors, but I always consider any form of arthritis as a serious sign that the spine has been under stress for several years. Although arthritis is common, it is not a diagnosis in and of itself. Instead, spinal arthritis is something to be seen on an x-ray, indicating that there is a problem. It often shows up as claw-like bony spurs, loss of space between vertebrae, poor alignment of one vertebra in relation to another, or narrowing of the foramen where the nerve exits.

Spinal arthritis or spinal decay is a sign of dysfunction and can be prevented. It is not inevitable nor is it age-related. I have seen hundreds of elderly patients with no signs of degenerative changes on their x-rays, and I have encountered just as many 30 year olds with advanced changes on theirs.

The cascade of events that cause spinal decay has been well documented by the eminent Drs. Kirkaldy and Willis, as well as Dr. Panjabi. It has become accepted in the medical community that the formation of bony spurs in the spine is in fact a response to abnormal motion or dysfunction in a spinal joint. These spurs, which until recently were written off as "arthritis," are actually a sign that the body, in its infinite wisdom, is attempting to stabilize a dysfunctional joint by the only way it can—through the laying down of more bone.

As with most spinal disorders, chiropractic care is effective in the treatment of degenerative joint disease. By restoring and maintaining movement to spinal joints through chiropractic manipulation, the physical effects (loss of motion, stiffness, etc.) to those with spinal arthritis may be kept to a minimum or prevented altogether. Rehabilitation and home exercises prescribed by your chiropractor will help keep the stabilizing spinal muscles strong and flexible to prevent further problems. In many cases, nutritional advice or dietary considerations may be helpful.

LEG LENGTH INEQUALITY "SHORT LEG SYNDROME"

Having one leg shorter than the other is like driving a car with two different tires. Low back, hip, knee, or leg pain can be caused by such a disorder, which may go undetected for years. Leg length inequality is often discovered by a variety of means used by chiropractors. These include x-rays, manual postural leg checks, and measurements on a patient with a tape measure.

A 1983 study published in *Spine* showed that only 43.5% of a control group had more than a 5mm leg length discrepancy, whereas over 75% of people with chronic low back pain have one leg shorter than the other. Leg length inequality has the potential to cause problems over time through altered spinal biomechanics and abnormal weight bearing. This, in turn, can contribute to the potential for injury and prolonged recovery when other spinal problems exist.

Pre-existing or co-existing spinal problems such as leg length inequality, poor muscle tone, subluxations, or degenerative conditions often "set the stage" for spinal problems in the future.

In some cases, however, this problem is not the only reason for back pain and may have no significance whatsoever. For example, a small leg length discrepancy in an accountant with back pain while sitting at his disk is less of a concern than a large leg length difference in a marathon runner who experiences back pain while running. As a holistic practitioner, a qualified chiropractor will be able to look at the "big picture" and diagnosis whether or not this structural problem has any effect on your current health status. If he or she thinks that the inequality is an issue, custom foot orthotics may be prescribed along with a course of chiropractic adjustments and exercises to normalize spinal biomechanics.

The fact that muscular and structural distortions contribute to back problems is not lost on the medical profession. For example, in a 1996 article in *Spine*, Gordon Waddell, M.D. aptly pointed out that when disc herniations occur, they are often superimposed upon existing conditions such as dysfunction, degeneration, and deconditioning.

SACROILIAC SYNDROME

The sacroiliac joint (SI joint) consists of the sacrum (the triangle-shaped bone at the base of the spine) and the ilium (pelvic bone). This joint is the connection between the ground and your spine. It acts as a shock absorber, transmitting all the forces of the upper body to the hips, pelvis, and legs.

Dysfunction in the sacroiliac joint is thought to cause low back and occasional leg pain. Sometimes, the pain is similar to that of a herniated lumbar disc or facet joint disorder.

Treatment of pain emanating from the sacroiliac joint is based on an accurate diagnosis because the SI joint may become painful for two completely different reasons:

* The joint may not be moving or mobile. This is known as a hypomobility, fixation, or sacroiliac subluxation. This type of pain is often felt on one side of the low back, buttocks, groin, or leg just above the knee.
* The SI joint has the potential to move too much. This is referred to as hypermobility or instability.

In my office, hypermobile sacroiliac joints are often seen in pregnant patients with low back pain. Often, they are referred to me by their OB/GYN for natural and safe treatment. Because of hormonal effects on the sacroiliac ligaments that cause the relaxation of the pelvis for the birthing process, the SI joint can become too "loose." These ligaments, which "hold" the pelvic bones together, can become over-relaxed, causing the muscles of the pelvis, abdomen, low back, and hips to compensate, resulting in pain and spasm. These sacroiliac ligaments can also be torn by traumatic event such as a fall, accident, or lifting injury.

To make treatment more challenging, it is often the cause of SI joint pain that must be corrected before any long-term relief is obtained. Many patients in my clinic have undergone multiple treatments and sometimes-unnecessary surgery, for what turns out to be an SI joint disorder.

Chiropractic care has been the treatment of choice for sacroiliac syndrome for decades. Traditional physio-therapy (heat, ultrasound, etc.) has been shown to have mild effects on the healing process of SI syndromes. Braces and support belts may be used to temporarily stabilize the joint and allow the ligaments to heal (which can also be facilitated by nutritional support). However prolonged bracing may weaken the muscles around the joint, so a transition to a supervised program of chiropractic adjustments and exercise is important.

In many cases, abnormal biomechanics must be corrected before the SI joint dysfunction stabilizes. This is often done through Foot Levelers custom orthotics (which can correct leg length inequality, excessive turning of the feet, knees, or hips).

FAILED BACK SURGERY

The New England Journal of Medicine reported that surgery is overused in the treatment of back pain. (NEJM; 2001:344 (5) pp363-69).

Spinal surgery is not performed to literally "cut out" the patient's pain. It is an attempt to change anatomy and remove or change whatever tissue is the probable cause of the patient's pain.

Spinal surgery is only basically able to accomplish two things: 1) decompression a nerve that is being pinched or choked, or 2) stabilize a painful spinal joint.

There are reasons for spinal surgery, which we will discuss in Chapter 9. Certain spinal surgeries, such as microdiscectomy and spinal fusion, have a more favorable outcome than others. The key, however, is to make sure that a patient has exhausted all conservative options for care, and that the area to be operated on is, in fact, the pain-producing tissue. This is well beyond the scope of this book.

There are several causes of failed back surgery. Unfortunately, spinal fusion procedures have the potential to transfer motion to the level above the operation, which may speed up the degenerative process at the level and result in pain.

Lumbar decompression surgeries may result in recurrent disc herniation (which is seen in 5-10% of cases), inadequate decompression, or nerve damage that either occurs during surgery or does not heal after decompression. Sometimes, decompressing a nerve during surgery may temporarily inflame the nerve and result in pain until the inflammation subsides. Scar tissue may form around the nerve after surgery.

In general, if there has not been improvement in three months after a spinal surgery, the operation may be deemed unsuccessful; further diagnostic tests or treatment may be reasonable.

Treatment of failed back surgery is based on what part of the spine is causing the pain. Many chiropractors are train in the treatment of failed back surgery. These are often complicated cases and usually require a structured treatment program.

Stretching can help reduce scar tissue formation if it is done within 6 to 12 weeks after the surgery. Education on proper posture, body position, and movement is often helpful. Range of motion, strengthening, and exercise programs definitely have a role. In cases where another disc is causing pain, spinal decompression therapy may provide relief. When the sacroiliac or facet joints are painful, chiropractic adjustments may reduce symptoms and increase mobility. If the pain is coming from irritated or tight muscles or trigger points, soft tissue therapies have the potential to minimize the associated pain.

SPRAINS, STRAINS AND SPASM

Muscle pain is only thought to be the cause of 20% of all back pain. In most cases where there has been trauma or injury, the muscles around a degenerated, dysfunctional, or inflamed area of the spine are in spasm or tighten in an attempt to protect the area. In cases of direct trauma such as falls, car accidents, or sports injuries, there may be extensive damage to the soft tissues. When a tendon or muscle has been injured, it is called a "strain." If a ligament is injured, torn, or damaged, it is referred to as a "sprain." In most cases of spinal soft tissue injury, both the tendons and ligaments are involved. This is referred to as a "sprain-strain."

The role of chiropractic care in managing sprain-strain injuries to the muscles, tendons, and ligaments is based on relieving pain, promoting full tissue healing, restoration of function, reduction of the potential for re-injury, and prevention of accelerated spinal degeneration.

When an injury to the back or neck occurs, there are **four phases of healing** that the region must undergo. Qualified Doctors of Chiropractic have been extensively trained in specific treatment procedures and goals specific to each phase of healing.

PHASE 1: ACTIVE SWELLING

Within the first 12-72 hours of an injury, swelling occurs as cells center the area to prevent further damage. This often results in pain and loss of motion in the area. During this phase, your chiropractor will recommend rest and support of the area by taping, bracing, or other protective means. Ice is often used during this period to reduce pain and to minimize spasms and swelling.

PHASE 2: PASSIVE CONGESTION

The second phase of healing an injury is known as "passive congestion." This usually begins on the second to fourth day, and during this time the fluid in the injured area tends to become counterproductive, causing increased pain and loss of motion. Doctors of Chiropractic often use manipulation or mobilization during this phase to slowly restore movement to the region, resulting in pain relief and increased motion. Physiotherapy modalities and basic exercise may also reduce unnecessary congestion.

PHASE 3: REPAIR

Around the fifth day after an injury, scar tissue begins to form around the area. This is known as the repair phase and can continue for up to six weeks. Lack of motion during the phase of healing can be detrimental, and scar tissue may form excessively, resulting in stiffness, limited range of motion, and poor joint mechanics. If motion is restored and maintained during this phase, tissues will heal more functionally.

Chiropractic care should continue throughout the repair phase as chiropractic treatment can be effective in restoring motion and proper biomechanics, improving connective tissue alignment, preventing scar tissue shortening, and restoring normal muscular tone and coordination.

PHASE 4: REMODELING

The final stage of injury healing is known as the remodeling phase. This phase can take 3-14 weeks and sometimes up to a year to complete. During this time, connective tissue remodels to provide strength and flexibility around the area of injury. Chiropractic treatment continues to be useful during this final phase, as it assists in the continued improvement of motion and flexibility, maintenance of function, reduction of pain, and minimizing the risk of injury.

STRESS

Whenever you experience stress, your body responds by increasing your blood pressure and heart rate, flooding your body with stress hormones and tightening up your muscles. When you are constantly stressed, the chronic tension causes your muscles to become sore, weak, and loaded with trigger points and muscle tightness, which often results in imbalance. This can contribute to the subluxation, resulting in a vicious cycle of pain and spinal dysfunction. If you are constantly under stress and you have low back pain, it is important to do some relaxation exercises, such as deep breathing, and getting regular physical exercise.

CHAPTER 3

Neck and Upper Back Pain

"The power that made the body heals the body."

BJ Palmer, Son of D.D. Palmer,
Pioneer of Chiropractic

While not as common as low back pain, neck pain affects almost everyone at some point in his or her life. Although most causes of neck pain are not due to severe traumatic injury, the pain can be just as disabling whatever the cause. In my office I am seeing an increase in neck pain more so than any other condition. With so many jobs, requiring patients to sit at a computer for eight hours a day, I for see the problem only becoming worse in the years to come. This poor posture leads to stress on the joints, muscles, ligaments and bones and it is only a matter of time before you start suffering from neck pain. People do not realize how much they move their neck during the day until they are unable to do so. The degree of flexibility of the neck, coupled with the fact that it has the least amount of muscular stabilization and it has to support and move your 14-16 pound head, means that the neck is very susceptible to injury. You can picture your neck and head much like a bowling ball being held on top of a stick by small, thin, elastic bands. It doesn't take much force to disrupt that delicate balance.

As you read earlier, the spinal cord runs through a space in the vertebrae to send nerve impulses to every part of the body. Between each pair of cervical vertebrae, the spinal cord sends off large bundles of nerves that run down the arms and to some degree, the upper back. This means that if your arm is hurting, it may actually be a problem in the neck! Symptoms in the arms can include numbness, tingling, cold, aching, and "pins and needles." These symptoms can be confused with carpal tunnel syndrome, a painful condition in the hands that is often found in people who work at computer keyboards or perform other repetitive motion tasks for extended periods.

Problems in the neck can also contribute to headaches, muscle spasms in the shoulders and upper back, ringing in the ears, dizziness and vertigo, temporomandibular joint dysfunction (TMJ), restricted range of motion and chronic muscle tightness in the neck and upper back.

We will talk about the neck and upper back together, because most of the muscles associated with the neck either attach to, or are located in, the upper back. These muscles include the trapezius, the levator scapulae, the cervical paraspinal muscles and the scalene, as well as others. Another important concept to remember when talking about neck pain is that neck pain is often the result of a lack of flexibility and mobility in the thoracic region (middle back). If the middle back is not moving correctly and is very stiff and tight then neck has to compensate for the middle back. This compensation leads to increase demands on the neck and often leads to instability and ultimately pain.

THE CAUSE OF NECK AND UPPER BACK PAIN

Most neck and upper back pain is caused by a combination of factors including injury, poor posture, subluxation, stress, and disc problems.

POOR POSTURE

One of the most common causes of neck pain, and sometimes headaches, is poor posture. It's easy to get into bad posture habits without even realizing it—even an activity as "innocent" as reading in bed can ultimately lead to pain, headaches, and more serious problems. The basic rule is simple: keep your neck in a "neutral" position whenever possible. Don't bend or hunch your neck forward for long periods. Also, try not to sit in one position for a long time. If you must sit for an extended period, make sure your posture is good: Keep your head in a neutral position, make sure your back is supported, keep your knees slightly about your hips, and rest your arms if possible. Use a pillow that supports the natural curve of your neck sleeping.

Poor posture can cause more than neck pain and headaches. Poor posture and its affect on overall health was studied in 2005, when a group of medical doctors sought out to determine whether or not there was a correlation between health and a patient's head position as measures by x-rays. This study, published in the September 15th issue of *Spine*, look at 752 adult patients. These patients were x-rayed from the side, and measurements to determine posture were recorded and correlated with the patient's health status. Findings of this study clearly illustrated that patients with a forward head posture ("chin-poking") had deterioration of their health status, increased pain, and decreased function.

Because posture is so important, I have devoted an entire chapter section on it in Chapter 7.

CERVICAL DISC HERNIATION

The discs in your cervical spine can herniated or bulge and put pressure on the nerves that exit from the spine through that area. Although cervical discs do not herniate nearly as often as lumbar discs do, they occasionally can herniate such as when the discs sustain damage from an injury. When this happens, most people experience radiating pain, numbness, tingling, or burning in their upper back, shoulders, arms, hands and fingers. There have been some cases of pain that was initially diagnosed as a rotator cuff injury or carpal tunnel syndrome when, in fact, the problem was arising out of a herniated or bulging disc in the neck.

Spinal Decompression and spinal adjustments, when performed by a highly trained Doctor of Chiropractic, can be safe and effective treatments for cervical disc herniations. Chiropractors use a variety of tests and physical maneuvers on each patient to determine the appropriateness of treatment.

Chiropractic treatments of disc herniations in the neck are usually coupled with other physical treatments such as The McKenzie Method or other exercise protocols and soft tissue techniques to decrease spasms and pain. These techniques and procedures are discussed in Chapter 5.

A case series in 1997, published in *The Journal of Manipulative & Physiological Therapeutics,* revealed 80% of disc herniations treated with chiropractic care had a good clinical outcome, and 63% actually had a reduction in the size, or complete resolution (this means they disappeared), of the disc herniations seen on the MRI before the study began!

CERVICAL SUBLUXATIONS

Subluxation is commonly seen at the transitional areas of the spine, such as where the upper neck meets the skull, the middle of the neck (where mechanically stress is greatest), and in the region where the lower neck and upper mid-back meet. (Subluxation is discussed in detail in Chapter 2.)

Each of these subluxation areas are associated with particular symptoms. The upper most subluxations between the cervical spine and the skull tend to cause headaches. Subluxations in the middle of the neck tend to cause neck stiffness and pain. Subluxations at the transition between the cervical and thoracic areas of the spine tend to create chronic muscle tightness and trigger points in the trapezius and levator scapulae muscles in the upper back. Subluxations in the middle of the thoracic spine tend to lead to mid-back pain, as well as disease and dysfunction in those areas that receive innervation (nerve supply) form the nerves, which exit the thoracic spine.

As we have previously addressed, Doctors of Chiropractic are the only health care providers trained in detecting and treating subluxations.

CERVICAL DEGENERATIVE DISC DISEASE

Degenerative disc disease in the neck is similar to that in the low back, where we discussed in Chapter 2. Degenerative disc disease in the cervical spine can be responsible for causing neck pain, headaches, and pain, burning, or numbness in the shoulders and arms.

A 2002 article in *Spine*, which studied 68 patients with degenerative disk disease of the neck, compared spinal adjustments, rest, and flexion exercises of the neck to surgery. The study concluded that non-surgical care (such as that given by a Doctor of Chiropractic) of neck degeneration is equally as good as surgery.

Cervical spine decompression and exercise, two commonly used treatments for neck pain, were shown to be more effective than analgesics (pain medications) in a 2002 study published in the *Bangladesh Medical Resource Council Bulletin*.

WHIPLASH SYNDROME

By far, the most common injury to the neck is a whiplash injury. Whiplash is caused by a sudden movement of the head, either backward, forward, or sideways, that results in damage to the supporting muscles, ligaments, and other connective tissues in the neck and upper back. Whether from a car accident, sports, or an accident at work, whiplash injuries need to be taken very seriously. Too often people don't seek the necessary treatment following a car accident or sports injury because they don't feel pain. Unfortunately, by the time more serious complications develop, some of the damage from the injury may have become permanent. Numerous studies have shown that years after whiplash victims settle their insurance claims, roughly half of them state that they still suffer with symptoms from their injuries.

Injuries to the neck from trauma, such as motor vehicle accident or sports injury, are common and can be serious. If you have been in a recent car accident or suffered a whiplash injury from a fall or a sports injury take the time to get checked out by your local chiropractor.

CERVICAL FACET SYNDROME

Facet syndrome in the neck is similar to that in the low back, which is discussed in Chapter 2. When facet joints in the neck are locked up or irritated, you may experience a lack of motion, sharp pain when the bending your head back or sideways, or a general sense of stiffness in your neck. The pain may also extend into your upper back, shoulders, or upper arm. Facet joint pain rarely extends past the elbow.

According to the October 2005 edition of the *American Journal of Pain Management*, facet joints cause 54-67% of chronic neck pain. This article goes on to recommend adjustments, spinal decompression, and other treatments commonly used by Doctors of Chiropractic for neck pain.

As with low back facet disorders, chiropractic adjustments often improve motion in the facet joints and help to restore and maintain motion and flexibility in these joints. Exercises are often useful in improving function and preventing re-injury.

A 2002 article in *The Annals of Internal Medicine* suggested that manual (hands-on) therapy for neck pain might be more effective than physical therapy or conventional medical care for neck pain. In this study, 183 patients with neck pain were divided into three categories: 1) the first group underwent manual therapy for six weeks, 2) the second group underwent physical therapy, and 3) the third group was given advice on self-care from general practitioners. The results were as follows: *68% of patients who underwent manual therapy were completely recovered versus 50% of those who underwent physical therapy and 36% who received medical care.*

THORACIC OUTLET SYNDROME

Thoracic outlet syndrome (TOS) is a group of symptoms caused by the compression of blood vessels and nerves in the region where they exit in the lower neck and upper chest area. The nerves and vessels in this area, known as the thoracic outlet, can be compressed by spinal misalignment, skeletal abnormalities, or muscular or postural imbalance.

Care of this problem depends on the site of the compression, and usually involves a combination of chiropractic adjustments, manual soft tissue therapy, postural advice, and education, exercise to stretch and strengthen surrounding tissues, and other non-surgical treatments.

A WORD ABOUT STRESS

When most people become stressed, they unconsciously contract their muscles, in particular, the muscles in their back. This 'muscle guarding' is a survival response designed to protect against injury. In today's world where we are not exposed to physical danger most of the time, muscle guarding still occurs whenever we become emotionally stressed. The areas most affected are the muscles in the neck, upper back, and low back. For most of us, the particular muscle affected by stress is the trapezius muscle, where daily stress usually leads to chronic tightness and the development of trigger points.

The two most effective ways to reduce the physical effects of stress is to increase your activity level (exercise) and do deep breathing exercises. When you decrease the physical effects of stress, you can substantially reduce the amount of tightness and pain in your upper back and neck.

TREATING NECK AND UPPER BACK PAIN WITH CHIROPRACTIC

In order to achieve the goal of reducing or eliminating upper back and neck pain, it is necessary to re-establish normal posture, mobility, strength, and coordination of the spinal vertebrae, joints and muscles. Numerous studies conducted by universities and funded by the U.S. government have shown repeatedly that chiropractic adjustments are one of the most effective means of treating problems in the spine, especially in the low back and neck regions.

EXERCISES FOR YOUR NECK AND UPPER BACK

Because you have to support the weight of your head on top of your highly unstable neck, it is critical that your neck and upper back muscles be flexible and strong. It is important, however, that when you start exercising a particular muscle or muscle group, that is free from spasms or trigger points in order to avoid irritating the muscle tissue. There are a number of exercises and stretches for your neck and upper back listed later in this book. If you have not done these exercises before, be sure to start off slow and light, and build up the intensity over several weeks. This will help you to avoid injuries to your muscles while improving your health.

CHAPTER 4

Headaches

"A quiet mind cureth all."

Robert Burton

Headaches affect just about everyone at some point, and they can present themselves in many different ways. Some people only experience pain one part of their head or behind the eyes; some people experience a pounding sensation inside their whole head. Some people experience nausea while others do not. The pain itself may be dull or sharp and may last for anywhere from a few minutes to a few days. Fortunately, very few headaches have serious underlying causes, but those that do require urgent medical attention.

Headaches are common, but they are NOT normal. Although the International Headache Society has classified 129 different types of headaches, the most common headaches come from the muscles (muscle tension), blood vessels (migraines), spinal joints (cervicogenic), or systemic conditions, such as high blood pressure and diabetes.

MUSCULAR TENSION HEADACHES

Tension type headaches are the most common type of headache, affecting upwards of 75% of all headache sufferers. Most people describe a tension headache as a constant dull, achy feeling either on one or both sides of the head. A tension headache is often described as a feeling of a tight band or dull ache around the head or behind the eyes. These headaches usually begin slowly and gradually, often in the middle or toward the end of the day.

Tension headaches, or stress headaches, can last from thirty minutes to several days. In some cases, chronic tension headaches may persist for many months. Although the pain can at times be severe, tension headaches are usually not associated with other symptoms such as throbbing, nausea, or vomiting.

The most common cause of tension headaches is subluxations in the upper back and neck, especially the upper neck, usually in combination with active trigger points. When the top of the cervical vertebrae lose their normal motion or position, a small muscle called the rectus capitis posterior minor muscle goes into spasm. This small muscle has a tendon that slips between the upper neck and the base of the skull and attaches to a thin tissue called the dura mater that covers the spinal cord and brain. Although the brain itself has no feeling, the dura mater is very pain-sensitive. Consequently, when the rectus capitis posterior minor muscle goes into spasm and its tendon tugs at the dura mater, a headache occurs.

Another cause of tension type headaches comes from referred pain from trigger points in the sternocleidomastoid muscle (SCM) on the side of the neck. These are much more common in people who have muscle damage in the neck caused by a whiplash injury.

MIGRAINE HEADACHES

Each year, about 25 million people in the U.S. experience migraine headaches. About 75% of migraine sufferers are women. Migraines are intense, throbbing headaches that are often associated with nausea and sensitivity to light or noise. They can last from as little as a few hours to as long as a few days. Many of these who suffer from migraines experience visual symptoms called an "aura" just prior to an attack that is sometimes described as seeing flashing lights. Sometimes, it appears as though everything has taken on a dream-like appearance.

Migraine headaches tend to run in the families and most sufferers have their first attack before the age of 30, supporting the notion that there is a genetic component to them. Some people have attacks several times a month; others have them less than one time a year. Many people find that migraine attacks occur less frequently and become less severe as they get older.

Migraine headaches are caused by a constriction of the blood vessels in the brain, followed by a reflexive over-dilation. During the constriction of the blood vessels, there is a decrease in blood flow, which is what leads to the visual symptoms that many people experience. Even in people who don't experience the classic migraine aura, there is a sense that an attack in imminent. Once the blood vessels dilate, there is a rapid increase in blood pressure inside the head. It is this increased pressure that leads to the pounding headache. Each time the heart beats, it sends another shock wave through the carotid arteries in the neck up to the brain.

There are many theories about why the blood vessels constrict in the first place, but no one knows for sure. What we do know is that there are a number of things that can trigger migraines such as lack of sleep, stress, flashing lights, strong odors, changing weather patterns, and several foods—especially foods that are high in an amino acid called 'tyramine.' At the end of this chapter, I have listed a number of foods that are most likely to trigger migraines as well as some **lifestyle changes** that you can make to reduce the likelihood that you will trigger a migraine headache.

CERVICOGENIC HEADACHES

Headaches originating in the neck have been shown to be responsible for almost 20% of the headaches in patients who have more than five headaches per month. This type of headache impairs function and reduces quality of life as much, or more, than migraine headaches.

Patients with cervicogenic headaches are likely to have neck pain or tenderness in addition to the headache itself. These people often describe their pain as "piercing" or "dull." Their symptoms begin in the middle of the upper neck and can radiate into the sides of the head near the temples or behind the eyes. These headaches often become more severe once they radiate from the neck into the head and can last from hours to weeks. People with these headaches are likely to have impaired motion of the neck, often finding it difficult to bend the neck forward or rotate the head from side to side.

CLUSTER HEADACHES

Cluster headaches are typically very short-duration, excruciating headaches and are usually felt on one side of the head behind the eyes. Cluster headaches affect about one million people in the United

States and, unlike migraines, are much more common in men. This is the only type of headache that tends to occur at night. The reason that they are called 'cluster' headaches is that they tend to occur one to four times per day over a period of several days. After one cluster of headaches is over, it may be months or even years before they occur again. Like migraines, cluster headaches are likely to be related to an over-dilation of the blood vessels in the brain, causing a localized increase in pressure.

CHIROPRACTIC CARE FOR HEADACHES

Chiropractic treatment of headaches is very patient-specific but generally involves a two-step approach of non-pharmalogical treatments such as adjustments, soft tissue treatments, biofeedback, exercise and nutritional advice along with avoiding triggers that cause headaches in the first place.

Numerous research studies have shown that chiropractic adjustments are very effective for treating tension headaches, especially headaches that originate in the neck.

A report released in 2001 by researchers at the Duke University Evidence-Based Practice Center in Durham, North Carolina, found that "spinal adjustments resulted in almost immediate improvement for those headaches that originate in the neck, and had significantly fewer side effects and longer-lasting relief of tension-type headaches than commonly prescribed medications."

These findings support an earlier study published in *The Journal of Manipulative and Physiological Therapeutics*, which found spinal adjustment therapy to be very effective for treating tension headaches. This study also found that even those patients who stopped chiropractic treatment after only four weeks continued to experience a sustained benefit in contrast to those patients who received pain medication.

In 2003, a double-blinded, placebo-controlled study compared migraine patients undergoing chiropractic manipulation versus electric muscle stimulation. After only two months of treatment, the severity and frequency of migraine headaches were significantly less in the chiropractic patients. The patients receiving chiropractic care continued to have a measurable improvement in symptoms compared to the control group of two months after the treatments.

The Journal of the Neuormusculoskeletal System reported in 2002 that within nine chiropractic treatments, sufferers of tension-type headaches averaged 64% improvement in their symptoms.

Spinal adjustment involves a hands-on approach to restoring mobility to spinal joints in the neck and upper back and often helps to reduce nerve irritation and restore normal curvature in the neck, relieve muscle spasm, and improve circulation.

Several soft tissue techniques such as Active Release Techniques (ART) and Graston Technique are useful in the treatment of headaches. These techniques are use to release muscle tightness and spasms in the upper back, neck, and in the suboccipital area at the base of the skull. The suboccipital area, in particular, has been implicated in most tension or cervicogenic headaches, which is why many patients report feeling their headache begins in their neck or back of the head.

Each individual's case is different and requires a thorough evaluation before a proper course of chiropractic care can be determined. However, in most cases of tension headaches, significant improvement is accomplished through adjustments to the junction between the cervical and thoracic spine. This is also helpful in cases of migraine headaches as long as food and lifestyle triggers are avoided as well.

AVOID HEADACHE TRIGGERS

* Stress may be a trigger, but certain foods, odors, menstrual periods, and changes in weather are among many factors that may also trigger headaches.

* Emotional factors such as depression, anxiety, frustration, letdown, and even nervous excitement may be associated with developing headaches.

* Keeping a headache dairy will help you determine whether factors such as food or changes in weather and/or mood have any relationship to your headache pattern.

* Repeated exposure to nitrite compounds can result in a dull, pounding headache that may be accomplished by a flush face. Nitrites, which dilate blood vessels, are found in such

products as hot dogs, sausage, brats, bologna, and other processed meats.

❋ Eating foods prepared with MSG can result in headaches. Soy sauce, meat tenderizer, and a variety of packaged foods contain this chemical, which is touted as a flavor enhancer.

❋ Headaches can also result from exposure to poisons such as insecticides and herbicides. Children who ingest flakes of lead paint may develop headaches.

❋ Foods that are high in the amino acid tyramine should also be avoided, such as ripened cheese (such as cheddar or brie), chocolate, as well as any pickled or fermented foods.

CHAPTER 5

Chiropractic Care

"The doctor of the future will give no medicine but will interest his patients in the care of the human frame, in diet and in the cause and prevent of disease."

Thomas Edison

WHAT IS CHIROPRACTIC?

Chiropractic is a branch of the healing arts that focuses on the relationship between structure and function in the human body. The term *chiropractic* comes from the Greek words *cheiro* and *praktikos*, meaning "done by hand." The purpose of chiropractic treatment is to uncover the cause of your symptoms, not to merely cover up these symptoms.

Doctors of Chiropractic do not prescribe medications or perform surgery. Rather, they draw from a wealth of training and resources to treat patients through conservative (non-invasive) treatments. Chiropractic care is aimed at restoring and maintaining normal structure and function of the joints, muscles and nervous system.

CHIROPRACTIC IN THE 21ST CENTURY

Once thought of as "alternative" or "complementary" to traditional medical care, chiropractic treatment has, over the past decade, become part of the mainstream health care. Over 15 million people utilize chiropractic care, and chiropractors are seen in private practice, within hospitals, and in multidisciplinary clinics throughout the world.

Doctors of Chiropractic serve on insurance boards, teach in prominent medical schools, and testify as experts in forensic cases. Chiropractic has become integrated into the modern healthcare system and is, in fact, more recognized and accepted than many other nontraditional therapies. **Chiropractors are an integral part of a health care team in the 21st century and are an invaluable resource in the non-operative treatment of pain.**

THREE PHASES OF CHIROPRACTIC CARE

Chiropractic care following an injury is like building a house—certain things have to happen in a particular order for everything to stand. When building a house, if you tried to put up your walls before you had a solid foundation, your walls would be weak and eventually collapse. If you tried to put on your roof before the walls were ready, you would run into the same problem. The same is true for your body, which has to go through a particular plan of care in order to repair itself correctly and fully. There are three general phases of chiropractic care: 1) relief care, 2) corrective care, and 3) maintenance care. How long each phase of care takes depends on the severity of the injuries.

PHASE ONE—RELIEF CARE

Many people go to a chiropractor because they are in pain. In this first phase of care, the main goal is to relieve you of your symptoms. Sometimes this will require frequent treatments. If you are in pain when you come to our office, the first objective is to help you feel better. Depending on the severity of your problem, it is typical to be treated three times per week for 4-6 weeks.

Most people are under the assumption that they don't feel any pain that there is nothing wrong with them—that they are healthy. Unfortunately, pain is a very poor indicator of health. In fact, pain and other symptoms frequently only appear after a disease or other condition has become advanced. For example, consider a cavity in your tooth. Does it hurt when it first develops or only after it has become serious? How about heart disease? Regardless of whether you are talking about cancer, heart disease, diabetes, stress, or problems with the spine, pain is usually the last thing to appear. When you begin chiropractic care, pain is also the first symptom to disappear, even though much of the underlying condition remains.

PHASE TWO—CORRECTIVE CARE

Most chiropractors regard the elimination of symptoms the easiest part of a course of treatment. If all the chiropractor does is to remove the pain and stop there, the chances of the condition recurring are much greater. In order to avoid a rapid recurrence of symptoms, it may be necessary to continue treatment even though your symptoms are gone.

During the corrective care phase, muscles and other tissues are allowed to heal more completely, thereby helping to prevent re-injury. It is typical to be treated two times per week for four weeks, during this phase of care as your body continues to heal.

During the correction phase of your treatment, you will not be treated as often as you did during the first phase of care and, depending on your particular circumstances, you may begin doing exercises and stretches at home to help accelerate your healing. Do not be discouraged if your symptoms include mild flare-ups on occasion... this is normal. Flare-ups are bound to occur during the corrective phase because your body has not fully recovered. Depending on the severity of your injury or condition and how long you have suffered from it, this phase of your care usually lasts 4-6 weeks.

PHASE THREE—MAINTENANCE CARE

Once your body has fully healed, routine maintenance chiropractic care can help ensure that your physical problems do not return, and keep your body in optimal condition. Just like continuing an exercise program and eating well in order to sustain the benefits of exercise and a proper diet, it is necessary to continue chiropractic care to ensure the health of your musculoskeletal system. When you make routine chiropractic care a part of your lifestyle, you can avoid many of the aches and pains that so many people suffer.

Once your body has fully healed, it is important to come in for periodic adjustments to avoid problems in the future. Usually, this only requires a quick visit to the chiropractor about once a month or so.

COMMON FORMS OF TREATMENT USED BY CHIROPRACTORS

Chiropractors use a variety of techniques and procedures in the treatment of spinal problems and for the promotion of overall health and wellness. The most commonly used methods of treatment in my office are discussed in this chapter. As with any healing art, the type of treatment is based on a variety of factors that assessed when a history is taken and the patient is examined.

CHIROPRACTIC ADJUSTMENTS

Perhaps the most common treatment associated with chiropractic is the use of chiropractic adjustments. This procedure is sometimes referred to as chiropractic manipulative therapy or "adjustments" because the spine is being "adjusted" to create movement and restore its range of motion. **The objective of a chiropractic adjustment is to reduce subluxation, which results in increased range of motion, reduced nerve irritability, and improved function.**

During an adjustment, a trained Doctor of Chiropractic manually administers a small, quick thrust into a spinal joint. This may be associated with a cracking or popping sound, which has been shown in research studies to be a release of small pockets of air bubbles (oxygen, nitrogen, and carbon dioxide) within the spinal joint. The sound is simply a release of gas, similar to opening a can of soda. The sensation with a chiropractic adjustment is usually one of relief.

Contrary to popular belief, a chiropractic adjustment is not an attempt to fix a "bone out of place." In the early days of chiropractic, the "bone out of place" model was used to explain the concept of subluxation and should not be taken literally. (*Subluxation has been discussed in Chapter 2.*) It is important to remember that the spinal joints that are functioning properly are not painful and are less likely to become injured or degenerate.

Scientific evidence of the effectiveness of chiropractic adjustments has been demonstrated over and over. It has been proven to be effective in treating mechanical disturbances in the spine, and may have wider positive effects on health and wellness.

Again, we look to sound research studies to illustrate what chiropractic adjustments have been shown to do:

* **Increase the size of the spinal canal.** This provides more room for the spinal cord, and decreases the effects of spinal conditions that narrow this important space (such as spinal stenosis, degenerative disc disease, and facet syndrome). (*Journal of the Neuromusculoskeletal System*, 1998)

* **Gap open the spinal facet joints** (A common source of pain the back and neck) as seen on MRI and studies at the National University of Health Sciences. (*Spine*, 2002; 2459-2466)

* **Increase range of motion in the spine.** Spinal joint range of motion increases with chiropractic treatment. This is especially important in cases of injury, trauma, or degenerative changes, which often cause loss of motion in the spine. (*Journal of Manipulative & Physiological Therapeutics*, 1992; 15:495-500)

* **Reduce spinal pain.** Chiropractic treatments have been shown to affect the levels of pain. (*American Journal of Physical Medicine*, 1984; 63:217-25)

* **Increase pain tolerance in spinal muscles.** These muscles, which are often effected with injury, degenerate disorders, disc problems, or subluxation, actually become more resistant to pain after chiropractic treatments. (*Journal of Manipulative & Physiological Therapeutics*, 1990; 13:13-16)

Reduce the electrical activity and tension in muscles. The
excitability of back muscles is decreased after a chiropractic treatment. This relaxation often eases pain and increases
function. (*Journal of Manipulative & Physiological Therapeutics*, 1987; 10:300-04)

Reduce blood pressure. Chiropractic treatments have been
shown to positively affect blood pressure. (*Journal of Manipulative & Physiological Therapeutics*, 1988; 11:484-488)

Increase plasma endorphins and melatonin levels. Mela-
tonin has been used to treat insomnia as well as boosting the
immune system. Endorphins are naturally occurring neurotransmitters that are analgesic, meaning they help alleviate
pain. The levels of these chemicals actually increase after a
chiropractic adjustment. (*Journal of Manipulative & Physiological Therapeutics*, 1986; 9:119-123)

Decrease the excitability and irritation of spinal nerves.
Chiropractic adjustments have been shown to reduce the
hyper-excited and irritable states of nerves. (*Spine*, 2000;
25:2519-25)

Down-regulate (decrease) inflammatory chemicals. In a re-
cent study, one chiropractic treatment to the thoracic spine was
shown to decrease plasma levels of pro-inflammatory chemicals (known as cytokines). (*Journal of Manipulative & Physiological Therapeutics*, Volume 29, Number 1; pages 14-21)

Research regarding the effects of chiropractic treatment is ongo-
ing and promising. Currently, studies on disabling diseases such as

asthma, multiple sclerosis, Alzheimer's, angina, and others are underway.

Although spinal adjustments are utilized by most chiropractors and is the treatment method most commonly associated with chiropractic, the mode of treatment is only one of many used by a chiropractor. In my office, for example, a variety of patient and condition-specific methods of treatment are utilized to get the most relief and correction in the least amount of time.

SPINAL DECOMPRESSION THERAPY

Spinal decompression is a non-invasive, non-surgical, safe and effective treatment for herniated discs, bulging discs, sciatica, numbness & tingling, annular tears, spinal stenosis, radiating pain down your leg or arms. Spinal decompression works by slowly and gently stretching the spine at a certain angle, taking pressure off the compressed discs and nerves. Spinal Decompression Therapy has shown great results for long-term pain relief.

Spinal decompression therapy has been shown to:
* Increase intervertebral disc height
* Reduce and eliminate herniated discs
* Eliminate bulging discs
* Remove tension in the pain-sensitive outer annular fibers of the disc
* Decrease the pressure within the inside (nucleus) of the disc
* Open and decrease the pressure around the spinal nerves
* Restore motion to spinal joints

In a 2005 study in the *European Spinal Journal,* this technique was shown to be more effective than exercise for patients with low back pain and sciatica. In my office, this treatment is often combined with exercises and produces dramatic results.

According to a 2002 article in *Neurosurgical Focus,* 75% of patients with neck and arm pain, muscle weakness, and loss of a reflex will respond to spinal decompression of the neck. Another 2002 article, this one in the medical publication *Radiology,* studied what happens to a cervical disc herniation during spinal decompression. The patients underwent an MRI while spinal decompression was applied to their neck. Eighteen of the twenty-one patients studied had partial reduction of their herniations, and actually three had complete resolution!

In addition, there are multiple published case studies showing a reduction of disc herniations and protrusions, decrease disc-related back and leg pain, and restoration of function with this technique.

EXPERT RESOURCE: To view a video on Spinal Decompression and to learn about this amazing technique visit: http://www.SpringfieldSpinalDecompression.com

MUSCLE MEDICINE

Manual therapy is a major focus of chiropractic care. Doctors of Chiropractic undergo a rigorous education in the evaluation and treatment of disorders associated with soft tissues.

Whether your injury or pain is in your lower back, neck, shoulder, hip, knee or even your feet, there is a good chance that part of the problem is coming from muscles. Muscles are an often an overlooked, important piece of any treatment plan. A sore shoulder, a tight lower back, or an achy knee in virtually everyone over the age of thirty, are common problems. They are often taken for granted as the inevitable consequence of getting older. But that's just not true. Whether a tight or injured muscle is the primary cause of pain and restriction or whether the main problem is inside the joints, the tools exist to get to the root of the problem.

ACTIVE RELEASE TECHNIQUES

One technique that is safe and highly effective at treating soft tissue injuries is called Active Release Techniques, or ART for short. ART is a patented, state of the art soft tissue system based massage technique that treats problems with muscles, tendons, ligaments, fascia, and nerves. Headaches, back pain, carpal tunnel syndrome, knee pain, shoulder pain, sciatica, plantar fasciitis, and tennis elbow are just a few of the many conditions that can be resolved quickly and permanently with ART. These conditions all have one important thing in common: **They are often a result of overused muscles.**

ART has been developed, refined, and patented by Dr. Michael Leahy. Dr. Leahy noticed that the symptoms of his patients seem to be related to changes in their soft tissue that could be felt by hand. By observing how muscles, fascia, tendons, ligaments, and nerves responded to different types of work, Dr. Leahy was able to consistently resolve 90% of the problems of his patients. Dr. Leahy came up with The Cumulative Injury Cycle. Dr. Leahy figured out that the over-used muscles results in weak and tight muscles. This then causes friction and tension on the muscle, which decreases the circulation, causing swelling (Edema). The decreased circulation and swelling lead to decreased oxygen called "hypoxia." Hypoxia in the muscles leads to the formation of scar tissue or adhesions in the muscles. The muscle adhesions then put additional stress on the muscles, making the muscles overworked, which lead to more injuries and pain.

A great example of this is how many people have gone to get a massage, and the massage felt great. Then, the next day or a few hours later, the muscle pain or tightness comes right back. In that case, the muscles probably have scar tissue and adhesions from repetitive trauma. The massages do not loosen up the scar tissue and adhesions, so as soon the massage is over, the problem comes right back.

In my office, I work closely with my massage therapists, because they recognize when a patient has muscular adhesions and scar tissue. They refer the patient to me for ART to fix the scar tissue and adhesions. Once we remove the adhesions, the patient then gets referred back the to the massage therapist for their normal massage.

The cumulative injury cycle is the affect that acute injury, repetitive trauma, and constant pressure or tension has on muscles, tendons, ligaments, nerves and bones. In the cyclic nature of an injury one factor triggers the next in a circular series. See the cumulative injury cycle below.

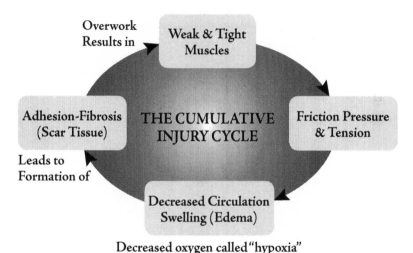

Overwork Results in → Weak & Tight Muscles

Adhesion-Fibrosis (Scar Tissue)

THE CUMULATIVE INJURY CYCLE

Friction Pressure & Tension

Leads to Formation of

Decreased Circulation Swelling (Edema)

Decreased oxygen called "hypoxia"

Copyright © 1995
P. Michael Leahy, DC, CCSO
Cumulative Trauma Disorder Defined

So, you might be asking how this overuse or repetitive strain conditions occur. Repetitive strain injuries occur from three different ways. They are:

* Acute injuries (such as pulls, tears, collisions, etc)
* Accumulation of small tears from micro-trauma (such as sitting on a computer for 8 hours a day)
* Not getting enough oxygen (hypoxia)

Each of these factors can cause your body to produce tough, dense scar tissue in the affected area. This scar tissue binds up and ties down the tissues that need to move freely. As scar tissue builds up, muscles become shorter and weaker, tension on the tendons causes tendonitis, and nerves can become trapped. This can result in the reduction of the range of motion, loss of strength, and pain. If a nerve is trapped, you may also feel tingling, numbness, and weakness.

A great example of this process is with carpal tunnel syndrome. **Did you know when the computer was invented there was a dramatic increase in carpal tunnel syndrome cases?** The reason why there was such an enormous increase in the amount of cases is because of the amount of recovery time.

Before computers, when people typed on typewriters, the recovery time between keystrokes was much greater. It took a longer amount of time for the key to be pressed down, resulting in a great recovery time for the muscles performing that action before the next key was pressed. Once the computer came around, the recovery time between keystrokes was significantly decreased. In the process, it has decreased the recovery time for the muscles, performing the action, thus, leading to more rapid repetitive motions.

As I sit here today, typing up this book on my Dell laptop, the amount of pressure needed to make a key stroke is much less, even compared to the first computers developed, and it is much quicker than a typewriter. Do you think the keyboards are going to be easier to type or harder to type on in the future? I think that we all know the answer to that question.

This decreased recovery time leads to repetitive motions that lead to an overuse injury in the muscle of the forearm. The muscles in your forearm are screaming for a break, but you just start work for the day. You have another seven hours to go. This nonstop, constant repetitive motion is what leads to muscle adhesions in the forearm muscles. And, as we just learned, this leads to tighter and tighter muscles. Eventually, the muscles are so tight that the tendon for the forearm muscles starts to get irritated and inflamed. The tendon becomes inflamed after awhile, and you'll start to develop elbow tendonitis (inflammation in the tendon). At this point in the cumulative injury cycle, the process continues to repeat itself until, finally, one day, one of the nerves that supplies the hand, "the carpal tunnel nerve", starts to become trapped under the tight muscles in the forearm. As the nerve gets trapped under the muscle, any time you use the muscle, the nerve gets more and more irritated and inflamed. Once the nerve becomes irritated and inflamed, you start to develop numbness and tingling in your hand. You have just developed… Carpal Tunnel Syndrome.

This is a very common scenario that I see daily in my office, ranging from carpal tunnel syndrome, sciatica, neck pain, or a herniated disc. Most musculoskeletal pain has some muscular component to the pain syndrome.

So, you might be wondering, what is ART treatment like? Every ART treatment is actually a combination of an examination and a treatment. The ART doctor uses his or her hands to evaluate the texture, tightness and movement of muscles, fascia, tendons, ligaments and nerves. Abnormal soft tissues are treated by combining precisely directed tension with very specific patient movements.

There are over 500 different treatment protocols unique to ART. This allows the providers to identify and correct the specific problems that are affecting each individual patient. ART is a safe and highly effective treatment for a variety of musculoskeletal conditions.

GRASTON TECHNIQUE

A second technique that is safe and highly effective at treating soft tissue injuries is called the Graston Technique. The Graston Technique is a patented form of instrument-assisted soft tissue mobilization technique that enables doctors to effectively break down muscle adhesions, scar tissue, and fascia restrictions. This technique utilizes specially designed stainless steel instruments to specifically detect and treat areas of soft tissue fibrosis or chronic inflammation, such as tendonitis. Since many long-standing spinal problems produce inflammation, muscle changes, and fibrotic scar tissue, this approach is helpful in creating significant, long-term changes to soft tissues throughout your body.

The handheld instruments that are used allow for a deeper, more sensitive palpation and treatment of restricted tissues. Since the metal instruments do not compress like the fat pads of the fingers, deeper restrictions can be accessed and resolved. Plus, their concave/convex shapes mold to the various contours of your body for greater comfort and effectiveness.

Originally developed for the treatment of athletic injuries, patients reported excellent results with both acute and chronic soft tissue injuries. The Graston Technique has resolved 87% or more of all conditions treated. It is equally effective on restoring function to acute and chronic injuries and pre- and post-surgical patients.

Graston Technique helps to:
* Decrease recovery time
* Reduce the need for medications
* Resolve long-standing conditions

Excellent results have been reported with injuries to the:
* Muscles
* Tendons
* Ligaments
* Fascia

This work will often resolve a number of common health complaints:
* Headaches
* Back pain
* Carpal tunnel syndrome

* Shin splints
* Shoulder pain
* Sciatica
* Plantar fasciitis
* Knee problems
* Tennis elbow
* IT Band Syndrome

Most of these conditions share one important common denominator: **overused muscles.** We use this technique, because it's a proven, state-of-the-art soft tissue system that helps many muscle-related conditions resolve quickly and permanently.

GRASTON TECHNIQUE
Chiropractors often use traditional physiotherapy modalities to assist in treatment to speed and enhance healing.

ICE THERAPY
Ice has long been used to treat many painful conditions and is most often used to reduce swelling and help control pain immediately after an injury and throughout the inflammatory stage. When ice packs are applied, they can decrease the temperatures of the surrounding tissues by 10-15 degrees, slowing down the metabolism in the tissues and reducing inflammation and pain.

Cold applied to the area decrease the flow of fluid into the tissues and slows the release of chemicals that cause pain and inflammation. Cold decreases feeling in an area by reducing the ability of the nerve endings to conduct impulses. The pain-relieving effect of ice results from decreased firing of the pain nerves and a relaxation of the muscle fibers. Cold also decreases the activity of cells, which works to reduce swelling and internal bleeding at the site of an acute injury. Cooling the deep tissue also reduces muscle spasm by reducing the muscle's ability to maintain a contraction.

HEAT THERAPY

Heat therapy involves the application of hot packs to the surface of the skin in an effort to heat the underlying tissues. The warmth decreases muscle spasm, relaxes tense muscles, relieves pain, increases blood flow and can increase range of motion. However, because heat can also increase inflammation in an injured area, it is important to never use heat therapy during the initial acute stages of an injury when inflammation is at its worst.

Heat therapy is most effective when used in conjunction with an active exercise program and it can be used effectively as part of a home care program under the supervision of a chiropractor.

THERAPEUTIC ULTRASOUND

Therapeutic ultrasound is a form of deep heat therapy created by very high frequency sound waves, hence the name ultra-sound. These sound waves are a form of micro-massage that helps reduce swelling, increase blood flow, decrease pain, and speed healing. Ideally, ultrasound treatment should begin immediately after a trauma and may be administered daily. It has been shown to reduce the inflammatory period and thereby accelerate the healing process. During the repair stage, ultrasound can stimulate the development of the capillaries necessary to re-establish a healthy blood supply to the damaged area.

One of the greatest benefits of therapeutic ultrasound is in the later stages of healing where the primary goal of therapy is to increase soft tissue flexibility. The deep heating effects of ultrasound make the muscle more pliable and, when combined with stretching, ultrasound is very useful for increase the range of motion in the neck and upper back.

ELECTRIC MUSCLE STIMULATION

Today, there are a number of different electrical stimulation (EMS) therapies available, all with their own particular benefits. Some are more beneficial for pain relief or to reduce inflammation, some for muscle spasm, and some actually cause muscles to contract in order to reduce muscle atrophy. In general, this type of therapy transmits light electrical pulses through the skin and into specific areas of the body.

Interferential therapy is a unique type of electrical stimulation that is very effective in decreasing pain and muscle spasm, and is very helpful during healing. One of the greatest benefits of interferential therapy is its ability to prevent the development of myofascial pain syndromes during the initial stages of healing after an injury when the muscles are the most vulnerable. It can be useful in promoting soft tissue healing and the restoration of muscle strength. The use of interferential therapy can dramatically improve the rate and degree of recovery and is often used in our clinic for acute pain.

EXERCISE

No treatment program for pain is complete without involvement of the patient in his or her care. Although many therapies are passive (administered to you by a doctor or therapist), it is the active (patient-guided) tools that cannot be neglected or underemphasized. The success or failure in correcting a spinal problem rests largely on your determination to play an active role in your care.

Because of its safety and effectiveness when used appropriately, exercise is a main area of focus in most chiropractic offices. I spend a great deal of time designing exercise programs, explaining exercise techniques, and guiding patients through rehab programs.

Exercise and rehabilitation programs should not be "cookie cutter;" every patient is different. Your specific condition, level of fitness, areas of improper function or deconditioning, and other factors need to be considered when your doctor or therapist prescribes an exercise program for you.

Many patients ask me to provide them with a strengthening program using weights or machines to perform at the gym in order to make their back stronger after an injury. Their train of thought is that some type of weakness is responsible for causing pain. Often, however, weakness in the spinal muscles is not the issue. Rather, weak abdominal muscles, and deep spinal muscles that rotate or flex the spine, or an imbalance between the spinal and abdominal muscles is the problem. For such patients, stronger abdominal muscles or a core stability program will offer a better outcome than a strengthening program of weight lifting for the muscles in the back.

Another example, The McKenzie Method, is an exercise protocol commonly prescribed for patients with low back pain and tends to emphasize extension (bending backwards) as part of the routine. Although effective for many types of back pain, these exercises may not be recommended for people with spinal stenosis, spondylolisthesis, and certain facet syndromes.

The wrong type of exercise programs can prolong recovery or even increase the risk of injury. Doctors of Chiropractic are well trained in detecting muscular weakness and patterns of imbalance in the human body, and many chiropractors have extensive experience and post-graduate training in McKenzie Therapy, Spinal Core Stability & Multifidus exercises or other forms of spinal exercise and rehabilitation therapy.

Remember, every treatment protocol for back or neck pain should have some type of exercise component. Prehab (preventative rehabilitation) exercises, exercises that may help in preventing back and neck pain, are presented in Chapter 7. For a more detailed or thorough program, seek care with your local chiropractor.

KINESIO TAPING

Proprioception refers to the body's ability to sense movement within joints enabling you to know where our limbs are in space without having to look. For example, if you stand on one leg and you feel your ankle rock back and forth, and shake this is challenging the proprioception in your ankle. The proprioceptive system is made up of special nerves in the muscles, joints, and ligaments that can sense tension and stretch and pass this information to the brain.

When a part of the body is injured, there is often a disruption in the proprioceptive system, resulting in a loss of normal sensation and coordinated movement. This can leave you prone to re-injury and decrease your performance if you are involved in a sport.

One simple way of re-establishing normal proprioception in a damaged area of the body is with kinesio taping. Kinesio taping involves placing strips of tape across an injured area in an attempt to brace or over stimulate the nerves in the area. This allows the brain and nervous system to develop normal coordination and restore function. You may have seen kinesio tape in action during the Beijing Olympics, when gold medal winner Kerry Walsh and Misty May used the "black tape" on their shoulder injuries.

The kinesio tape can be worn for 4-5 days at a time, in the shower or during a workout, with no problems. Although it is mostly used with athletes, it can also be used to treat neck injuries and lower back injuries as well. To learn more about kinesio taping please visit http://www.kinesiotaping.com/

SPINAL PELVIC STABILIZER CUSTOM ORTHOTICS

Many chiropractors prescribe custom foot orthotics for patients. In cases where there is a leg length discrepancy or foot disorder contributing to altered biomechanics in the pelvis and spine, orthotics play a role in stabilizing the region "from the ground up." Think of it in terms of a house. If the foundation of a house is off the rest of the house is going to be off kilter. Just like the foundation of the house if your foundation, your feet, is not leveled, the rest of the body is going to be out of alignment.

Results from a 2003 study suggest that custom-made Spinal Pelvic Stabilizers custom orthotics help improve body balance while standing. Studies in 1996 and 2002 in the *Journal of Manipulative & Physiological Therapeutics* and *The Journal of Sports Chiropractic and Rehabilitation* have shown that Spinal Pelvic Stabilizers from Foot Levelers Company may help improvement alignment, function, performance, and gait (walking).

In my office we digitally scan each patient's feet to look at the arches of their feet to determine if their "foundation" is level. We have seen patients suffering from knee pain, hip pain, lower back pain, and even neck pain resolve with the use of Spinal Pelvic Stabilizers orthotics. To learn more about Foot Levelers go to http://www.footlevelers.com/

NUTRITIONAL SUPPORT

Proper nutrition is vital during the process of healing and recovering from an injury. In addition, many recent dietary recommendations and nutritional supplements decrease inflammation or slow the progression of degenerative spinal disorders. Doctors of Chiropractic are on the few health care providers who stress nutrition and diet in treating and preventing disease. We will discuss nutrition in more detail in Chapter 8.

COLD LASER THERAPY

Albert Einstein wrote a theory about lasers in 1917, and the laser was invented in 1960. Laser light is monochromatic (one color), coherent (all wave are in phase with each other), and can be collimated (meaning held to a small spot size at a great distance).

Lasers work by penetrating through your skin and are absorbed by special components in your body's cells called *chromophores*. Just as photosynthesis creates energy for plants, the absorption of the photons by your cells causes increased production of cellular energy. In areas of injury or damage, this means there is more energy available to improve the rate and quality of healing. This is called *biostimulation*.

For patients, this means relief from acute and chronic pain, reduced inflammation and muscle spasms, improved range of motion and restored function. Patients suffering from headaches, neck pain, carpal tunnel, low back pain, sports injuries, post-surgical pain, and more have been helped with laser therapy.

Some patients notice improvement after the very first treatment session; with others it may take a few treatments. The effect of the laser therapy is cumulative, meaning that each successive treatment builds on previous ones. Cold laser therapy produces a mild, soothing, warm feeling. You may notice a tingling sensation in the treatment area as the blood vessels dilate, or that muscle spasms are reducing in strength and duration. Laser therapy is a painless treatment. Laser therapy is a painless treatment. To learn more about laser therapy go to http://www.klasers.com/

CHAPTER 6

Frequently Asked Questions

"The only true wisdom is in knowing you know nothing."

Socrates

Q: Once you see a chiropractor you have to go for the rest of your life?

How long you decide to benefit from chiropractic care is always up to you. As I have stated previously, many conditions respond quickly and require minimal care programs and in office protocols usually lasting three months in duration. There is, however, mounting evidence that preventative or maintenance care is effective.

For example, in 2004, a study in the *Journal of Manipulative & Physiological Therapeutics* sought out to determine whether or not chiropractic care is able to actually prevent back pain flair-ups.

The author studied 30 patients who suffered from back pain for at least six months. All patients underwent twelve chiropractic treatments over the course of one month. Then, half of the patients did not undergo any further chiropractic care for nine months, while the other half continued care once every three weeks for the nine-month period.

At the end of the nine-month period, both groups were examined again. The authors found that both groups had a reduction in their pain during the entire study period. However, the patients undergoing chiropractic care experienced a significantly greater reduction in disability than the patients who did not continue care.

In my office most my patients choose to come in every 3-6 weeks for their chiropractic maintenance care. They have found it helps keep them pain free and prevent future injuries. Again, the choice is completely up to you.

Q: Are chiropractors real doctors?

Chiropractors are licensed as medical health care providers in every U.S. state and dozens of countries around the world. The chiropractic and medical school curricula are virtually identical. In fact, chiropractors have more hours of education than their counterparts. As part of their education, chiropractic students also complete approximately nine hundred hours of work in a clinical setting, assisting licensed chiropractors. Once chiropractic students graduate, they have to pass four sets of national board exams as well as state board exams in the states they want to practice.

Chiropractors receive extensive training, combined with many hours of practical work. Just like conventional medical doctors, chiropractors are medical professionals that are subject to the same testing, licensing, and monitoring by state and national peer-reviewed boards. Federal and state programs, such as Medicare and Workers' compensation programs, cover chiropractic.

The biggest difference between chiropractors and medical doctors lies not in their education or diagnostic ability but in their preferred method of treatment. Medical doctors are trained in the use of medications (chemicals that affect your internal biochemistry) and surgery. Consequently, if you have a chemical problem such as diabetes, hypothyroidism, or an infection, medical doctors can be very helpful. However, if your problem is mechanical or physical, there is no chemical in existence that can fix it. You need a physical treatment to correct a physical problem. That's where chiropractic care is at the forefront. **Chiropractors use physical treatments—adjustments, exercises, stretches, physiotherapies—to treat conditions that are physical, rather than chemical, in origin such as back pain, injuries, disc problems, muscle spasms, headaches, and poor posture.**

Chiropractic School Hours Vs. Medical School Hours

D.C.	SUBJECT	M.D.
540	ANATOMY—EMBRYOLOGY	508
240	PSYSIOLOGY	326
360	PATHOLOGY—GERIATRICS—PEDIATRICS	401
165	CHEMISTRY	325
120	MICROBIOLOGY	114
630	DIAGNOSIS—DERMATOLOGY EYES, EARS, NOSE, THROAT	324
320	NEUROLOGY	112
360	RADIOLOGY	148
60	PSYCHOLOGY—PSYCHIATRY	144
60	OBSTRETICS—GINECOLOGY	148
210	ORTHOPEDICS	156
3,065	TOTAL	2,706

(Based on the average the curriculum of 18 chiropractic colleges and 22 medical schools)

Q: Do chiropractors work with medical doctors?

Absolutely. At my office, I work hand-in-hand with medical professionals everyday. Personally, I enjoy working with primary care physicians, pain specialists, and spine surgeons in an attempt to get the best outcome for my patients. I communicate regularly with medical doctors, both to keep them informed on the status of their patients, and to offer my input on difficult cases. Patients benefit when there is open communication between health care providers, and this is encouraged in my office.

When a doctor refers a patient to my office for care, I take the trust they have placed in me by sending their patient to be both a great compliment and a great responsibility.

Q: How do I find the right chiropractor?

Finding a good chiropractor is like finding a good dentist. It is often useful to ask friends, co-workers, and neighbors for their recommendations. Primary care physicians or other health care providers may also be helpful. Generally speaking, if many resources recommend the same chiropractor, there's a good chance that he or she is reputable.

Also, with sites like Google and Yelp! You can read what other patients have to say about that chiropractor.

General questions that you may want to ask when seeking a Doctor of Chiropractic include:

* Have they completed the National Boards?

* How many years have they been in practice?

* Does the doctor have post-graduate training or advanced certification in any specific treatment or method? For example, I specialize in Active Release Techniques, Graston Technique, Rehabilitation and Spinal Decompression.

* Will the doctor stay in communication with my other health care providers?

* Do they belong to any reputable associations, academies, or societies?

Avoid doctors who recommend lengthy (more than 4-6 months) pre-scheduled treatment plans. Each patient is different, and no doctor can predict how much treatment you will require in year. Many patients do require extensive chiropractic care, but this is a decision that must be made as the care progresses, not at the first visit or several months in advance.

Q: What is a chiropractic adjustment?

A chiropractic adjustment is a gentle, quick thrust to a particular joint, typically in the spine, intended to restore normal position and movement. Adjustments are important for releasing adhesions in the joint and reducing stress on the nervous system. Because of the fact that the nervous system is the master controller of all muscles and organs in the body, removing stress on the nervous system through chiropractic adjustments will frequently lead to improved health in the entire body.

Q: Do chiropractic adjustments hurt?

Usually not. There have been some patients of mine that have experienced mild soreness after being adjusted, but this is more the exception. Most people feel better very quickly after being adjusted.

I often describe to patients that it may feel as if you had a really good workout tomorrow. On average, about 10% of my patients are sore.

Q: How many adjustments will I need?

The number of adjustments you will need depends on several factors including: your age, your overall health, and the extent of degenerative changes, de-conditioning, or spinal distortion.

If you are young, in good health, and have a mild condition that occurred very recently, you will need far fewer adjustments that if you are older, in poor health, and have been struggling with a problem for many years. The total number of adjustments you will need depends on whether you are merely interested in reducing the pain you are currently experiencing, or are interested in creating optimal long-term health.

Q: I have heard that chiropractic neck adjustments can cause you to have a stroke?

Strokes are definitely serious events, no doubt, and with any medical procedure there are certain risks. The risk of suffering a stroke from a chiropractic adjustment is extremely small, about the risk of being struck by lightning. In fact, you are 70,000 times more likely to suffer a stroke from the daily use of aspirin to prevent heart attacks than to suffer a stroke from a chiropractic adjustment. You are 37,000 times more likely to suffer a stroke form an unknown reason than to suffer a stroke from a chiropractic adjustment. When administered by a licensed Doctor of Chiropractic, adjustments are extremely safe.

Statistically, the likelihood of a vertebral artery dissection (which can result in a stroke) is estimated to be 1 in 500,000 to 1 in 300,000. These complication rates are considerably less than any treatment modality (even aspirin) for spinal pain management.

The risk of suffering a fatal stroke from an adjustment of the neck is 0.00025%. The risk of having a stroke in the general public is 0.00057%. What does that mean? The risk of having a stroke "out of the blue" is higher than the risk associated with a stroke from an adjustment of the neck.

Doctors of Chiropractic are trained to diagnosis patients who are prone to this disorder and may order tests to rule out the risk of a stroke. When there may be a risk of vascular problems, chiropractic techniques are changed or modified to avoid such complications.

Q: Does insurance cover chiropractic care?
Today, roughly 90% of insurance plans available cover chiropractic care, including Medicare and Worker's Compensation. Also, your car insurance Medpay will cover chiropractic care if you were

involved in an accident. It is rare today to find insurances that do not cover chiropractic care. To find out if you have chiropractic care coverage call your insurance company or have the office of the chiropractor you would like to see call to verify your benefits.

Q: My insurance company covers chiropractic care, but the number of visits is limited. Why?

How many Tylenol, will you take this year? How many times will you slip or fall? How many times will you need to exercise or eat right to maintain a level of health? Can you honestly predict in advance how many of any treatment a patient will need in a one-year period? So, I don't know how insurance companies do it.

Many patients in my office suffer from degenerative changes, disc disorders, spinal disorders often require more extensive chiropractic treatment. Patients with disc disorders in the neck or lower back may require 12 weeks of treatment, and sometimes more, to minimize the risk of nerve damage and avoid surgery. For some reason, however, this fact eludes insurance companies who "ration" medical and chiropractic treatment to their consumers (also known as patients) in an attempt to cut costs and appease company stockholders.

In my opinion, the determination of the number of frequency of treatments should be left to the discretion of the treating doctor and is not the same for everyone. In addition, my opinion is that supportive or maintenance chiropractic care as a means of preventing a reoccurrence of symptoms and restoration of function is a patient and doctor-based decision, and should not be left to the discretion of an insurance carrier, whose primary interest is cost containment.

Q: Can pregnant women undergo chiropractic care?

Chiropractic care is a safe and effective treatment for back pain during pregnancy, affecting over 60% of pregnant women. Expecting women are referred to my office almost weekly by their OB/GYN or midwife for problems in the low back, pelvis, or legs. Because they must avoid many medications for the sake of a healthy baby, many women seek natural methods of care for their problem.

A January, 2006, article in the *Journal of Midwifery and Women's Health,* reported that chiropractic treatment is safe (no adverse effects were seen in seventeen cases studied) and effective in reducing pain intensity associated with pregnancy.

Q: Do Doctors of Chiropractic prescribe medication?

Currently, chiropractors do not prescribe medications, although they may refer someone to another provider for prescription medication if it is deemed necessary. In most cases, however, patients are better off with physical, rather than chemical, treatments for physical problems.

We know that a chiropractic adjustment is safer than taking an aspirin. We also know that masking the symptoms with drugs usually does nothing to actually solve the underlying problem and that long-term use of narcotic pain medications carries with it the potential to cause addiction and drug dependence.

I am far from "anti-medication." I personally believe that there are times when medication has short-term use in managing back pain. However, long-term medication use for controlling back pain can be dangerous.

Q: Why is routine chiropractic care so important?

Many health-conscious adults go to the chiropractor for overall wellness and preventative measures. Chiropractic was originally founded on the premise that a properly functioning nervous system (for which the spine is the conduit from the brain to every organ and cell in the body) is vital for the expression of health.

Dr. Christopher Kent, in his testimony before the Senate Appropriations Committee, cited an insurance database analysis comparing chiropractic patients over 75 years old with patients of the same age who weren't seeing chiropractors. The data presented showed that the chiropractic patients reported better overall health, spent fewer days in nursing homes, used fewer prescription drugs, and were more active than the group of non-chiropractic patients.

In 1999, the *New England Journal of Medicine* shows us that chiropractic patients use 56% fewer anti-inflammatory drugs, 75% fewer muscle relaxants, and 98% less physical therapy in the management of their pain.

In 2000, a survey of 311 chiropractic patients, aged 65 and older, who had received chiropractic maintenance care for at least five years was reported in *The Journal of Manipulative & Physiological Thera-peutics*. These patients, compared to those not undergoing chiropractic care, spent 31% less than the national average for health care costs. They saw health care providers, on an average, half as often. They used less prescription drugs and less tobacco than their non-chiropractic counterparts.

In 2004, a health survey of 2,818 chiropractic patients from 156 clinics was published in the *Journal of Alternative & Complimentary Medicine*. This survey revealed that 95% of patients felt that their expectations had been met under chiropractic care, and 99% wished to continue care. In addition, there was a strong correlation between persons receiving chiropractic care and self-reported improvements in health, wellness and quality of life.

As previously mentioned, research is currently being done on the positive effects of chiropractic care beyond that of back pain. Clinical trials have shown promising results in other areas, and Doctors of Chiropractic have long been advocates for a Wellness Lifestyle, addressing such factors as diet, emotional well-being, rest, nutrition, and exercise.

CHAPTER 7

Prehab:
Exercises To Prevent

*"Opportunity is missed by most people because it is
dressed in overalls and looks like work."*

Thomas Edison

THE FOUNDATIONS OF SPINAL HEALTH

As we have discussed in the previous chapters of this book, the human body is an amazingly complex system of bones, joints, muscles, and nerves, designed to work together to accomplish one thing: movement. Everything about the human body is designed with movement in mind—nerve fibers stimulate the muscles to contract, muscles contract to move the bones, bones move around joints, and the nervous system controls it all.

As a matter of fact, research has shown that movement is key to our body's health that a lack of movement has a detrimental affect on everything from digestion to our emotional state, immune function, our ability to concentrate, how well we sleep, and even how long we live. The bottom line is that if your lifestyle does include enough movement, then your body cannot function efficiently. Consequently, three things will happen. First, you will not be as physically healthy and will suffer from a wide variety of physical ailments, ranging from headaches to high blood pressure. Second, you will not be as productive in your life because of reduced energy levels and the ability to mentally focus. Third, because you have less energy, your activity level will tend to drop off even further over time, creating a downward spiral of reduced energy and less activity until you get to a point where even the demands of a sedentary job leave you physically exhausted by the end of the day.

FOUNDATION ONE: POSTURE

The most immediate problem with poor posture is that is creates chronic muscle tension, as the weight of the head and upper body has to be supported by the muscles instead of the bones. This effect becomes more pronounced the further your posture deviates from your center of gravity.

To illustrate this idea further, think about carrying a briefcase. If you had to carry a briefcase with your arms outstretched in front of you, it would not take long before the muscles of your shoulders would be completely exhausted. This is because carrying the briefcase far away from your center of gravity places undue stress on your shoulder muscles. If you held the same briefcase down at your side, your muscles would not fatigue as quickly because the briefcase is closer to your center of gravity and the weight is, therefore, supported by the bones of the skeleton, rather than the muscles.

Correcting bad posture and the physical problems that result are accomplished by doing two things. The first is to eliminate as much 'bad' stress from your body as possible. Bad stress includes all the factors, habits, or stressors that cause your body to deviate from your center of gravity. This can include having a poor adjusted workstation, not having your seat adjusted correctly in your car, or even carrying too much weight around in a heavy purse or backpack.

The second is to apply 'good' stress on the body in an effort to move your posture back toward your center of gravity. Getting your body back to its center of gravity by improving your posture is critically important to improving how you feel. This is accomplished through a series of exercises, stretches, adjustments, and changes to your physical environment that all work to help correct your posture.

FOUNDATION TWO: MOVEMENT

Imagine waking up one morning with a frozen shoulder where you couldn't move your upper arm more than a few inches in any direction. How much would that impact your ability to do your job? How much would that affect your ability to drive your car or even dress yourself? How much would that affect your ability to concentrate on anything other than the shoulder? Obviously, if your shoulder did not move correctly, it would have a dramatic impact on your life. The same is true with movement in every part of your body. If things aren't moving the way they are supposed to move, it will have a negative impact on your ability to function at work and take care of the demands of everyday life, including your ability to concentrate.

Over the years, I have had a number of patients come into my office with severe low back pain who stated that their pain came on suddenly when they did something as simple as bend down to pick up the newspaper. Just about everyone would agree that a person's body should be able to handle something as simple as bending over to pick up a newspaper or putting on their socks, right? So what happened?

In every one of these cases, I have found that many of the joints in the body where barely moving at all; they were hypomobile or locked up. When the joints in one area of the body do not move the way they should, other areas of the body are forced to move more than they are were designed to in an effort to compensate for the area that is not moving. This creates significant stress on the areas that have to pick up the slack of the joints that aren't moving properly. This can lead to pain and inflammation. At the same time, those joints without normal movement can continue to stick together, causing the ligaments and tendons to shorten. This leaves the body in an unstable condition, and if left unchecked, can progress until the body can hardly move at all. This will cause the person to suffer flare-ups of pain at even the slightest provocation.

Most of us have seen people who have lost most of their normal mobility. This is especially prevalent among the elderly. Contrary to popular belief, this is not the inevitable effect of aging; rather it is the unfortunate effect of not maintaining the body's mobility through exercise, stretching, healthy alignment and body mechanics. There are a lot of people in their 60s, 70s, or even older, who are stronger and more flexible than the average person in their 30s simply because they keep themselves strong and flexible through exercise. Maintaining mobility is critical in order to live free from pain and disability. Maintaining good mobility is not difficult, but it does not happen on its own.

Just as in developing good posture, it is necessary that you perform specific exercises and stretches to keep your muscles, tendons, and ligaments flexible and healthy. In addition, it is crucial that all of the joints in your body move properly. Although this can be achieved to a great degree through the stretches described in this book, most people also find routine chiropractic adjustments to be very beneficial.

FOUNDATION THREE: STRENGTH

Strong muscles keep your body upright and allow you to move. Good muscle strength and balance are critical for proper posture and minimizing muscle tension. Your muscles function much like the wires that hold up a tall radio or television antenna. If the wires are equally strong on all sides, the antenna will stand up straight. If one of the wires becomes weak or breaks, the antenna will either lean to the side or collapse. The same is true with your body. If the muscles on the all sides of your spine are balanced and strong, your body will stand up straight and strong. Unfortunately, most people don't have balanced and strong muscles. The reason for this gets back to the lack of exercise and abnormal motion of the spine.

Muscles are very efficient at getting stronger or weaker in response to the demands placed on them. Since most of us sit at a desk, drive a car, and sit on the sofa at home, many of our muscles are not challenged. Consequently, they become weak. At the same time, the muscles that are constantly used throughout the day become strong. This imbalance of muscle strength contributes to poor posture and chronic muscle tension. Left unchecked, muscle imbalances tend to get worse, not better, because of a phenomenon called Reciprocal Inhibition.

Reciprocal Inhibition literally means, "shutting down the opposite." Simply put, for all of the muscles that move your body in one direction, there are opposing muscles that move the body in the opposite direction. In order to keep these muscles from working against each other, when the body contracts one muscle group, it forces the opposing group to relax—essentially shutting down the opposite muscles.

This phenomenon is especially important to people who work at a desk because all day long the same muscles in the upper back and chest area of the body are used. This means that throughout the day, the body is essentially shutting down the opposite muscles in the middle back. Over time, the muscles in the middle back become very weak because they are not being worked like the muscles in the front. This contributes to poor posture and chronic muscle spasm and pain.

The easiest way to correct this imbalance is to learn and perform specific exercises, which will increase the strength of the back muscles, along with manual therapy and chiropractic care. Once the muscles in your middle back are strong, the resultant tightness and poor posture often disappear.

FOUNDATION FOUR: COORDINATION

Healthy coordination is the result of using the body in the manner in which it was designed. Exercises such as walking, swimming, rock climbing, Yoga, Pilates, bicycling, martial arts, and strength training all help to improve muscle coordination, whereas working at a desk, reading, and watching television do the opposite.

Without realizing it, most people are in a dramatic state of muscle imbalance. This occurs simply because they sit for many hours every day and do not perform exercises on a regular basis that will work to keep all of the muscles in their body properly coordinated. This muscular imbalance contributes to muscle tightness, restricted movement, and joint pain.

THE IMPORTANCE OF EXERCISE

Everyone knows that exercise is important for good health. Study after study has shown that exercise is effective at decreasing pain, reducing stress, improving immune function, lowering blood pressure, improving cardiac function, boosting energy, improving sleep, and maintaining a healthy body weight. The fact remains that although most people are aware of how important exercise is to their health, they still do not exercise the way that they should. Another prime example of this is flossing your teeth. People are aware of the benefits of flossing and yet people often do not have the time for it. Really? You don't have the time for it, it takes about one minute to do and costs about 1 cent per day. The same goes for exercise, you need to exercise daily even it is just for 20-30 minutes. You need to examine your life and prioritize, making exercise one of your top daily priorities.

You don't have to exercise as intensely as Lance Armstrong to enjoy the benefits of exercise. But you do have to get up and get your body moving at least five or six days per week, preferably doing a combination of aerobic exercise and strength training. This will help you not only feel better and have more energy, but will help to stabilize and strengthen your whole body.

TYPES OF EXERCISE

As a former personal trainer, I am a huge proponent of regular exercise. Research has shown that certain exercises may reduce your chance of back pain and neck pain. My patients are given a specific regimen of exercises while under my care, and the protocol is tailored towards their specific condition.

In this chapter, I will introduce you to basic exercise concepts. I will also how you several muscle stretches and exercises that, when performed regularly, can help you prevent muscular imbalances, weakness, and in coordination, that may lead to future spinal problems.

AEROBIC EXERCISE

Aerobic means "using oxygen" and aerobic exercises are those that utilize oxygen during the activity. Activity exercise trains the body to utilize the oxygen more efficiently and improves your overall cardiovascular fitness. Aerobic activities are those that are performed for an extended period of time at a low intensity. Examples of aerobic activities are biking, aerobic walking, swimming, running, in-line skating, aerobic dance, cross-country skiing, and using an elliptical trainer. The benefits of aerobic activity include:

* Improved breathing
* Increased energy throughout the day
* Improved hearth health and cardiac output
* Decreased blood pressure
* Decreased cholesterol
* Decreased stress
* More restful sleep
* Improved mood and mental functioning
* Improved digestion and bowel function

For maximum benefit, you should engage in at least 30 minutes of aerobic activity five or six days per week. If you already do more than this, great! For those who have not engaged in regular activity for a while, even 30 minutes a day will be a significant accomplishment.

During aerobic exercise, you should be able to carry on a conversation without feeling too winded. If you are breathing too heavy while carrying on a conversation, you should ease up a bit. As you become healthier, you will be able to increase the intensity of your activity without feeling short of breath.

This brings up another important point—a concept called **the Overload Principle.** The Overload Principle simply states that in order to benefit from physical activity, the intensity has to be greater that what your body is used to. Only by pushing your body a little bit—by overloading it—will your body respond by growing stronger.

STRENGTH TRAINING

Strength training differs from aerobic training in three important ways. First, strength training involves activities that are more intense and much shorter in duration than aerobic activity, for example doing push-ups or sit-ups. Second, aerobic training primarily improves the health of your muscle, joints, and bones. Third, while aerobic activity should be performed almost every day for maximum benefit, you only need to engage in strength training two to three times per week in order to maximize the effects of training. The benefits of strength training include the following:

* Increased muscle and bone strength
* Improved muscle tone and body shape
* Improved hormone function
* Improved mood and mental functioning
* Decreased cholesterol
* Decreased stress
* More restful sleep
* Increased metabolism

To benefit from strength training, it is not necessary that you spend long grueling hours in the gym every day. In fact, you can experience a significant improvement in your strength and muscle tone by weightlifting for one hour, just two or three times a week!

The key to successful strength training is not the amount of time you spend; it is the intensity that is important. The harder you work your muscles during the strength workouts, the quicker you will see improvements. Each time you exercise your muscles harden, your body goes to work to build more muscle. As long as you continue to slowly increase the weight that you use week after week, your muscles will continue to grow in strength. Most people begin to see a difference in their strength and how they look after a few weeks of strength training.

STRETCHING

Stretching not feels great; it is also very effective at reducing muscle tension, decreasing stress, and maintaining flexibility and joint mobility. In order to experience the benefits of stretching, however, it is important that you stretch correctly. Stretching your muscles too hard, bouncing while holding a stretch, or stretching your muscles when they are too cold can injure your muscles and lead to muscle tightness. Proper stretching techniques are easy, provided you follow a few simple rules.

The first rule is to never stretch your muscles too hard. You should only stretch to the point where you feel a mild pull on the muscle. If you attempt to stretch further, you may cause small tears and create a reflex tightening of the muscle. Repetitive overstretching can cause scarring of the muscle and a loss of flexibility.

The second rule is to never bounce while stretching. When you bounce, you momentarily force your muscles to overstretch and increase the risk of muscular injury.

The third rule is to only stretch your muscles when they are warm. Muscles are a lot like plastic. If you heat plastic, you can bend it and stretch it without it breaking. By stretching once you are warmed up, stretching will be much more safe and effective.

THE MAGNIFICENT SIX:
EXERCISES TO PREVENT BACK AND NECK PAIN

The following exercises should be done at least every other day. They should be performed in the exact order shown, as I have designed the program to strengthen and stretch the key spinal muscles.

When starting this or any exercise program, please note the following:

Always check with your doctor before starting any exercise program. Stop the exercise if you are experiencing any discomfort or pain. Remember, these stretches and exercises are meant to create flexibility and strength, so minor discomforts from these movements is normal. Ease into your exercise program. Start slow, and add repetitions or sets as you progress.

Exercise 1: Abdominal Bracing

Lay on your back, with your knees bent and feet flat on the floor. Slowly rotate your pelvis, flattening your spine against the floor. As you do this, gently "brace" your stomach, as if someone is about to punch you in your stomach, while at the same time tightening your buttock muscles. Hold this position for 5 seconds and 10 repetitions.

Exercise 2: Glute Bridges

While still on your back, keep your spine straight (not arched), and tighten your stomach muscles while pushing down on your heels and slowly raising your buttocks off the floor. Hold this position for 5 seconds and repeat 10 times.

Exercise 3: Cat/Camel

Now, roll over to a comfortable position on the floor with your hands directly below your shoulders and your knees directly under your hips. Slowly tuck your chin and tighten your stomach muscles as you arch your back like a cat. Hold for a count of 5. Then slowly allow your stomach muscles to relax and let your mid-back sag. Repeat this cycle, arching and sagging, for a total of 10 repetitions.

Exercise 4: Side Plank

To perform a side plank, lie on your side and prop yourself up with your forearm. Your lower arm should be straight out from your side, with your hand in a fist. Use your opposite hand to grasp your shoulder to keep it steady. Hold your body like a plank with your hips, pelvis, and chest in a straight line and firm as a single unit.

First, focus on simply holding the position with good form, and then work toward 3 sets of 10-second reps on each side. To add difficulty, aim for more repetitions instead of longer durations. (Your body does not learn to stiffen when exhausted.) To add complexity, roll your torso as a block to alternate sides. Fast repetitions of torso turns make the exercise more difficult. Make sure that you roll with no spinal movement or rising of the hips.

Exercise 5: Curl Up ("The New Sit-Up")

To perform a curl up, lie on your back with one knee bent, your hands under your lumbar (lower back) curve, and your elbows lifted off the ground. Consciously pause to first stiffen your abdominal muscles. Then, brace your abdominals as if someone is about to punch you in your stomach. Then lift your head and neck together from the breastbone and lift up about 1" off the ground. Don't poke your chin forward. Hold for 7 or 8 seconds, breathing steadily, with your abs braced. Do as many as you can without losing your form.

If you experience neck pain, make sure that your head and neck come up together as a unit. Another trick, if you are still experiencing neck pain, is to press your tongue up against the roof of your mouth. This will engage the deep neck muscles, which should have been working during this exercise, and prevent neck pain.

Exercise 6: Bird Dog

Use this exercise to build a box of muscle around your midsection and strengthen the multifidus muscle in your low back. To perform this exercise, start out on your hands and knees. Before starting this exercise and throughout this exercise, make sure you brace your abdominals as if someone is about to punch you in your stomach. Extend one arm and opposite leg and hold this pose for 10 seconds. Next, extend the opposite arm and opposite leg and hold this pose for ten seconds. That is one repetition. Complete 9 more repetitions, for a total of 10 repetitions. As you get stronger, work up to doing 3 sets of 10 repetitions.

Throughout this exercise, it is critical that there be no motion in your back. You should be able perform this exercise with a yardstick on your back without falling off.

3 GREAT DAILY NECK EXERCISES

These daily exercises can be easily performed at home or your workplace, and are often useful as a "stress breaker."

Exercise 1: Levator Scapulae Stretch

Sitting comfortably, grasp the side of your chair, while with your right hand gently tilt and pull your head to the right. Hold this stretch for 5 seconds. Repeat this 5 times on the right, and then switch to the left. Repeat the exercise.

Exercise 2: Neck Stretch

Rest your left hand on your left shoulder blade. Turn your head to the right, and using your right hand gently pull your head in a diagonal direction until a gentle stretch is felt. Hold for 5 seconds.

Repeat the stretch on the opposite side. Perform a total of 5 stretches per side.

Exercise 3: Chest Stretch

Stand in an open doorway and place your hands at shoulder level on the doorframe. Slowly lean forward until you feel a gentle stretch across your chest and front shoulders. Hold for 5 seconds and repeat 5 times.

EXPERT RESOURCE:

To see videos on how to perform all of these core exercises and many more visit

http://www.NovaChiroWelllness.com/ExerciseVideos

CHAPTER 8

Nutrition

*"Each patient carries his own doctor inside him.
They come to us not knowing that truth.
We are at our best when we give the doctor who
resides in each patient a chance to work."*

Albert Schweitzer, MD

F ood is not simply an energy source for the body. Each piece of food you put into your mouth contains hundreds or thousands of individual chemicals that influence a wide range of functions, emotional state, and even your body weight. It is important to understand how carbohydrates, proteins, and fats influence your body's biochemistry so that you can make informed choices about the foods that you eat. Once you understand some simple ideas about food, you can use this knowledge to improve your overall health. In this chapter, you will learn how your body uses the three basic types of food—carbohydrates, fats, and proteins. You will also learn about certain vitamins, minerals, and herbs that are critical to your overall health.

CARBOHYDRATES

Carbohydrates are the main fuel source that your body uses to think, run, walk, breathe, and perform just about every action. Next to water, carbohydrates are the most consumed nutrients in the world. There are three types of carbohydrates that you consume every day: sugars, complex carbohydrates, and fiber.

In order for the body to use sugars and starches in food, it must first break them down to a form that can be used by your body's cells. The first step of the digestion process occurs in your mouth by an enzyme called salivary amylase. This enzyme begins the process of breaking down starches into simple sugars. Once the food reaches your stomach, the digestion of carbohydrates stops. It begins again once your food leaves the stomach and enters the small intestine.

The main purpose of the digestion process is to convert the carbohydrate you consumed into a simple sugar called glucose. Glucose is the primary fuel source for the brain, central nervous system, and nearly every other cell in your body.

To ensure a readily available supply of glucose, the body stores it in the muscle and liver in a form called glycogen. Glycogen is then converted back to glucose any time your blood glucose level drops too low. If you body uses all its glycogen, it will start breaking down muscle in order to provide your vital organs with the glucose they need to function.

The two major hormones that help regulate the level of glucose in your blood are insulin and glucagon. Insulin is a hormone that is released when your blood glucose levels rise, which typically occurs after you consume foods containing carbohydrates. The function of insulin is to signal the liver and muscle cells to remove the excess glucose from the blood and store it as glycogen.

Glucagon has the opposite effect. When your blood glucose levels become too low, glucagon will signal the muscle to convert glycogen back to glucose and release it into the blood stream. The balance of these two hormones helps to keep blood glucose levels within a fairly narrow range.

There are some instances where the body is unable to maintain healthy blood glucose levels. The most common condition is called diabetes and is caused by a loss of normal insulin function. Those with diabetes have abnormally high blood glucose levels. A much rarer condition called primary hypoglycemia is when blood glucose levels are abnormally low.

Not all carbohydrates have the same effect on the blood glucose levels. Starches are much larger molecules than sugars and therefore take longer to break down and enter the blood stream as glucose. Sugars, on the other hand, are simple molecules that can quickly be converted into glucose and enter the blood. Sugars will tend to create a sharp spike in blood glucose levels, whereas starches will tend to cause a much more gradual increase.

The measure of a food's ability to elevate blood glucose levels is referred to as its glycemic index. Simple sugars have a high glycemic index because they cause a very rapid increase in blood glucose levels. Larger, more complex carbohydrates such as starches have a low glycemic index because they cause a gradual increase in blood glucose levels.

High glycemic index foods—foods that contain a lot of sugar—will tend to increase your storage of body fat. The reason is that each fat cell in your body can also respond to insulin, take glucose of the blood, and store it. But instead of storing the extra glucose as glycogen like the muscles and liver do, it stores the excess glucose as fat. The higher your blood glucose rises, the more it will be stored in your fat cells. To minimize the amount of carbohydrates that ends up being stored as fat, it is important that you consume low glycemic index foods such as whole grains and pastas.

Carbohydrates are an essential part of any healthy diet, especially when you are on a weight loss program. It is important to stick to the low glycemic index carbs to avoid elevating your blood glucose to the point where the carbs end up being stored as fat.

PROTEINS

Proteins are required to maintain the normal structure and function of the body. Whereas carbohydrates, especially glucose, are the primary fuel source for the body, proteins are used as primary building blocks of the body tissues such as muscle, bone and connective tissue. In addition, the enzymes, antibodies, hemoglobin, and even your DNA are all made from protein.

Proteins are made up of about twenty different amino acids. Twelve of these amino acids can be synthesized in your body and, therefore, do not need to come from your diet. These are called the non-essential amino acids. The other eight amino acids are essential amino acids and need to come from your diet including isoleucine, leucine, lysine, methionine, phenylalanine, threonine, tryptophan and valine. If you do not get enough of these amino acids in your diet, your body cannot repair itself, your immune system can't do its job properly, your metabolism will decrease, and you will tend to feel sluggish, depressed, and tired. The primary source of these amino acids are from protein sources such as meat, fish, cheese, eggs, soy, dairy products, beans, and legumes.

Before your body can use the protein in your in food, it must first break down the protein to individual amino acids. Digestion of protein begins in the stomach where acids and proteolytic enzymes begin the process of release amino acids from the protein. Some amino acids are absorbed directly through the stomach lining and enter into the blood stream. The remaining protein then enters the small intestine where digestion is completed.

Once the amino acids enter the blood, the body can use them to build red blood cells, muscle tissue immune factors, or whatever else the body needs. However, all twenty amino acids must be present in the blood in the proper ratios in order for the body to manufacture new proteins. If one amino acid is missing or is present in a very limited quantity, then that amino acid becomes the limiting factor to protein synthesis. For this reason, it is best to eat proteins that have all of the amino acids that the body needs.

Proteins have an added advantage in that they don't cause a rapid increase in blood glucose levels, which makes them low glycemic index foods. In addition, proteins will increase your body's metabolism more than carbohydrates and fats and will provide building blocks for many mood-elevating neurotransmitters such as serotonin and dopamine.

Proteins are critical for building lean muscle tissue, and maintaining stable blood glucose levels, immune function, and normal brain chemistry.

FATS

Of the three major components of food, fats are certainly the most misunderstood. Fat is the not the bad thing that it is often made out to be. Your brain, spinal cord, and entire nervous system are largely made from fat as well as many of your hormones such as testosterone and estrogen. Fat provides your body with a store of energy and insulation from the cold, and it protects your organs from physical damage. In fact, next to water, fat is the most abundant substance in the human body, ideally averaging about 10%–20% of a person's total body weight.

Dietary fats are necessary for the proper absorption of fat-soluble vitamins, and scientists have recently discovered that some fats in the diet are used for sending signals to the brain to control how much to eat. It is not fats, per se, that you should avoid. You should only avoid eating too much of the wrong kind of fat, which is saturated fat.

Dietary fats come in several forms: saturated fats, polyunsaturated fats, monounsaturated fats, and cholesterol. Saturated fats are the demons of dietary fats because they can elevate blood cholesterol, leading to the development of heart disease. Saturated fats also tend to cause low-grade inflammation in the body. Animal fats are the most common source of saturated fat in the diet. Other sources are snack foods, which usually contain a lot of palm oil and palm kernel oil. You will want to avoid saturated fats whenever possible by selecting lower-fat meats such as chicken, turkey, and pork and avoid commercially prepared snack foods.

Polyunsaturated fats such as corn oil, flaxseed oil, or fish oil are much healthier forms of fat than saturated fats and tend to be liquid at room temperature, whereas saturated fats are usually solid. Unlike saturated fats, the polyunsaturates will help to decrease cholesterol, both LDL and HDL, and will help to decrease inflammation in the body.

Monounsaturated fats are even healthier for your body than either saturated fats or polyunsaturated fats. They not only decrease your bad LDL cholesterol, but they also help raise your good HDL cholesterol! Using olive oil, canola oil, avocados, and nuts in the preparation of your daily meals is the simplest way to introduce monounsaturates into your diet.

Cholesterol is a waxy fat that is found exclusively in animal foods—beef, chicken, fish, turkey, eggs, dairy, etc. Years ago it was believed that consuming cholesterol in your diet led to an increase in your blood cholesterol, but this turned out to be not the case. Dietary cholesterol has very little, if any, impact on blood cholesterol level of most people. The major negative contributors of cholesterol are eating too much saturated fat, being overweight, and not getting enough exercise.

CALORIES

A calorie is a measure of the energy content of food. Calories are what your body uses to keep your heart pumping, keep your lungs breathing, allow your mind to think, and give your muscles energy they need. Carbohydrates and protein each provide four calories per gram, fats provide nine calories per gram, and alcohol provides approximately seven calories per gram. In other words, ounce for ounce, proteins and carbohydrates give you fewer than half of the calories of fat. The high caloric value of fat is why high-fat foods such as cream cheese and fried foods are so high in calories. It is important to remember that calories are not your enemy. As strange as it may seem, if you don't eat enough food, it will be harder for you to lose weight because too much calorie restriction slows down your metabolism.

Maintaining a healthy body composition is a balancing act between calories you consume and the calories you burn. We have spent time discussing the main sources of energy in your diet—carbohydrates, proteins, and fats. Let's take a quick look at the other side of the equation—**how your body burns the calories you consume.**

Your body burns calories in two ways: your basal energy expenditure (also known as your basal metabolic rate) and your activity level. The biggest user of calories is your basal energy expenditure (BEE), which is the energy used by your organs to keep your body alive and to build muscles, bone, and connective tissue. Your BEE is responsible for burning up to three-fourths of all the calories you burn in one day.

Activity is the other way in which you burn calories. Depending on how active you are, activity can make up as little as fifteen percent or as much as thirty-five percent of the total calories you burn in a day.

NUTRITIONAL SUPPLEMENTS

I was recently told by a colleague that during a graduate nutrition course at the University of Minnesota, the professor posed a challenge to the class: *Construct a 2000 calorie-per day diet that at least met the Recommended Dietary Allowances (RDA) for vitamins and minerals without the use of supplements.* After all, we have always heard that if you eat a well-balanced diet, you don't need to take vitamin supplements, right? Well this professor was putting that statement to the test.

To everyone's surprise, no one was able to come up with a sustainable daily diet that met the minimum requirements for vitamin and mineral intake. The problem was not with getting the minimum vitamin intake; the challenge was getting enough of a few very important minerals, especially zinc. Unless you eat oysters or dark turkey meat every day, it is impossible to get the minimum RDA of zinc through diet alone.

The bottom line is that in order to get enough trace minerals in our diet to at least meet the minimum RDAs, it is necessary to take a good quality supplement.

Another argument for taking a multivitamin and mineral supplements is that there is substantial evidence that taking doses of a class of nutrients called antioxidants, which far exceed the RDA minimums, can help prevent heart disease, help to mitigate some of the detrimental effects of diabetes, and help to promote healthy immune function.

In today's environment, you will be hard pressed to find a health care provider who does not recommend a multivitamin. **I recommend all patients take a professional grade multi-vitamin, along with Vitamin D, Magnesium, and Omega-3 fish oil.** Those are the essential supplements everyone should be taking, according to the latest research.

4 ESSENTIAL SUPPLEMENTS TO SUPPORT YOUR ANTI-INFLAMMATORY DIET

Research continually supports the need to bolster a healthy diet with nutritional supplements to promote health and prevent disease. Inflammation reduction, antioxidant protection, and cellular health are mechanisms of many supplement products. The following supplements are recommended to promote a healthy inflammatory response and support specific nutritional needs:

* **Multivitamin and Minerals without Iron:**
The modern diet is known to be deficient in numerous micronutrients. Supplementation with a multivitamin/mineral can help address many of these deficiencies. Low micronutrient intake may accelerate the aging process and promote the diseases of aging and other chronic diseases. The use of a multivitamin is thought by many medical authorities to be a wise preventive strategy in addition to a healthy diet. Iron should only be taken by those who have an iron deficiency.

Vitamin D:

We derive virtually no vitamin D from a normal diet, and we are supposed to get vitamin D from the sun. Sunscreen with an SPF of 8 reduces vitamin D production by 95%. Subsequently, most Americans are chronically deficient in Vitamin D, which promotes a chronic inflammatory state that is associated with expression of numerous chronic diseases. Vitamin D deficiency is associated with chronic musculoskeletal pain, as well as numerous other diseases, including osteoporosis, osteoarthritis, fibromyalgia, autoimmunity, heart disease, cancer, diabetes, and depression. The addition of Vitamin D3 is designed to support cardiovascular health.

Magnesium:

Magnesium is chronically deficient in the modern diet and promotes a chronic inflammatory state. Magnesium deficiency is associated with diverse clinical manifestations, including heart disease, high blood pressure, diabetes, and headaches. Some researchers have recommended that magnesium be added to the water supply, because deficiency is associated with sudden death from heart disease, asthma, and neurological and psychiatric conditions. Magnesium plays a crucial role in glucose metabolism, cellular energy production (ATP), calcium transport, nerve signal condition, and over 300 reactions in the body.

Omega 3 Fish Oil (EPA/DHA):

Supplementing with omega-3 fatty acids addresses the deficiency of omega-3s in the modern diet and helps balance our ratio of omega-6 to omega-3 fatty acids. Adequate omega-3 intake helps to balance inflammatory activity and promote health. Adequate levels of omega-3 fatty acids help to promote joint and bone health, mental/emotional health, heart health, proper blood sugar regulation, nervous system health, and skin and eye health.

NATURAL MUSCLE RELAXANTS

In some cases, the use of natural muscle relaxants will be useful for spasm, sprains, muscles pulls, tension, soreness, or other muscle-related pain. Combinations of Boswellia extract, Tumeric, and Magnesium have been shown to be safe and may be effective for muscular pain and inflammation. I often give patients a combination of these natural ingredients, known as a Pain Recovery Pack.

A FINAL THOUGH ON NUTRITION

The foods you eat on a daily basis have a tremendous impact on your overall health. If you eat all-natural, health giving foods, your body will be healthy. If you eat junk, your physical health will suffer. Remember that your body's only source for its building materials is the food that you eat.

In addition to eating a wide variety of natural, health giving foods, it is also critical to take good quality supplements and drink plenty of water. The vitamin supplements ensure that all of the metabolic processes in your body can be performed effectively and the water helps to keep the metabolic waste and toxins flushed out of your system.

When clinically appropriate for specific conditions, the use of safe and natural supplements may speed healing, minimize inflammation, and reduce pain. The entire realm of nutritional management for specific health conditions is beyond the scope of this book and takes up volumes. Tumeric, Boswellia, and other Ayurvedic herbs are showing promise as strong anti-inflammatories. The use of homeopathic treatment in chiropractic offices is not uncommon. Preoteolytic enzymes may be useful in cases of acute injury.

As with any treatment recommendation, your doctor should be able to explain your nutritional options, as well as the latest research on the safety and effectiveness of anything he or she prescribes.

Conclusion

"Health is defined as a state of complete physical, mental, and social well-being, and not merely the absence of disease or infirmity."

The World Health Organization

Chiropractic care is about more than just treating back pain. As we have discussed, it is a holistic health care discipline that emphasizes wellness and prevention in addition to pain relief. By making the right lifestyle choices now, you have the potential to prevent health problems in the future.

The bad news is that nothing will guarantee that you will never suffer from back pain. However, exercising, eating well, getting plenty of rest, and not smoking will certainly go a long way toward keeping your back healthy and pain-free, but back or neck pain, like the common cold, seem to hit just about everyone at one time or another.

Now the good news: you can prevent most cases of back pain yourself with some simple stretches, exercises, and lifestyle changes. In fact, if you make these things a part of your daily routine, you can usually prevent back pain from occurring in the first place.

A NEW PARADIGM IN HEALTH CARE

Doctors have a responsibility to educate their patients, make recommendations based on solid medical evidence, and administer safe and effective therapies. However, true progress in the management of back pain not only involves treatments that are done to you (known as **passive treatment**) by a doctor or therapist, but also activities performed by you (known as **active care**).

Quitting smoking, following your doctor's advice, asking questions, losing weight, exercising, keeping scheduled appointments, eating a healthy diet, meditating, and learning about your problem and treatments is necessary for true progress.

I always emphasize the team approach between doctor and patient in managing back pain. My patients are confident that I will do all that I can provide them with quality care. In return, however, I expect positive lifestyle changes will enhance healing and overall wellness. True progress in managing back pain occurs when there is a synergistic formula of active and passive care.

Much like a finely tuned care, your body requires maintenance in the form of exercise, proper nutrition and diet, regular chiropractic adjustments, and positive lifestyle changes. By maintaining this "vehicle" now, you will minimize the need for more drastic interventions later.

When treatment for back pain is necessary, you can be confident that Doctors of Chiropractic are highly trained in diagnosis and management. The "team" of doctor and patient is broadened when various practitioners work together for the benefit of the patient.

By returning to this book as a reference in the future, you will possess an understanding of and an appreciation for the human body, and the spine in particular. You are now armed with a body of knowledge that will guide you in the pursuit of an **active, pain-free lifestyle.**

APPENDIX A: SPECIAL OFFERS

Consultation with Pain Severity Exam:
Valued Over $200.00

After reading *The Healthy Alternative: A Guide For A Pain- Free, Active Lifestyle* you may decide that you want to take action and stop living in pain and live a pain-free, active lifestyle that you deserve.

You don't have to wait any longer. You can work with Dr. Sullivan who will develop a treatment plan, implementing the techniques, exercises, nutritional changes and advice contained in this book.

The Healthy Alternative: A Guide For A Pain-Free, Active Lifestyle readers can request their **FREE first visit** to evaluate your condition, and to develop a treatment plan to get you on the road to living a pain-free, active lifestyle.

Call Today (703) 912-7822
To Schedule Your Appointment

*The free consult offered here does not apply to patients who participate in a federal program providing healthcare benefits or payments—such as, but not limited to, Medicare.

ABOUT THE AUTHOR

Dr. Todd P. Sullivan is the owner and clinic director of NOVA Chiropractic & Wellness Center in Springfield, VA. Dr. Sullivan received his Doctor of Chiropractic degree from New York Chiropractic College. Dr. Sullivan was one of two chiropractors selected to complete his residency training at the National Naval Medical Center (The President's Hospital) in Bethesda, MD. He is a sports chiropractor who specializes in the treatment of musculoskeletal injuries and people of all ages.

Dr. Sullivan has advanced training in treating soft tissue injuries that includes full certification in Active Release Technique (ART) and Graston Technique. He utilizes a functional approach combining therapies like Active Release Technique, Graston Technique, Chiropractic Joint Manipulation, Spinal Decompression, rehabilitation, and nutritional advice. Dr. Sullivan is also certified by Titleist Performance Institute in the diagnosis and treatment of golf injuries. He is a member of Professional Sports Care, which provides chiropractic care at PGA Tour events.

Dr. Sullivan has treated athletes from the NFL, NHL, MLB, NCAA, PGA and olympic athletes. He has also served on the medical staff at the IRONMAN World Championship in Kona, HI, National Marathon, Suntrust Marathon, and Cherry Blossom Ten Miler. Dr. Sullivan currently serves as the chiropractor for the Virginia Triathlon Series. An athlete all of his life he has experienced first hand knowledge of the benefits of sports chiropractic. Dr. Sullivan maintains an active lifestyle competing in marathons, triathlons, and golfing.

For more information about Dr. Sullivan's practice, to schedule a consultation, or to book Dr. Sullivan for a speaking engagement, you may contact his office at:

NOVA Chiropractic & Wellness Center
6230 Rolling Road, Suite J
Springfield, VA 22152
703-912-7822
toddpsullivan@gmail.com
NovaChiroWellness.com
SpringfieldSpinalDecompression.com

Made in the USA
Middletown, DE
19 April 2017